Regulatory
Biochemistry in
Neural Tissues

Regulatory Biochemistry in Neural Tissues

edited by
Louis Sokoloff

The MIT Press
Massachusetts Institute of Technology
Cambridge, Massachusetts

REGULATORY BIOCHEMISTRY IN NEURAL TISSUES

Introduction

LOUIS SOKOLOFF

A FEW WORDS ARE in order to define the nature and delineate the scope of the topic, *Regulatory Biochemistry of Neural Tissues*, as construed by us in the organization of the program. It will become obvious from the content of the presentations that the subject has been interpreted broadly and liberally to include extensive consideration of studies in biological systems other than nervous tissues. The choice has been deliberate. Years of study of the biochemistry of nervous tissues have led to the realization that basic biochemical processes in the CNS are not really fundamentally different from those of other tissues. Biochemical mechanisms elucidated first in simpler systems have in general been found to be quite relevant and to apply equally well to nervous tissues. The assumption has, therefore, been made that despite the unique functions of the nervous system, mechanisms of biochemical regulation in neural tissues will prove to be similar to those already defined or being elucidated in less complex cells and organisms. For this reason studies with all types of biological materials that contribute to the understanding of basic biochemical regulatory mechanisms have been accepted as being within the scope of this topic.

Biochemical regulation is currently a subject of intense interest and research activity. This wave of interest has evolved naturally and logically from the remarkable advances that have punctuated the history of biochemistry during the last several decades. Modern biochemistry was founded primarily in the old disciplines of physiological chemistry, euphemistically known as "blood and urine" chemistry, and nutrition. In its early period emphasis was placed on gross energy metabolism as studied by direct and indirect calorimetry and oxygen consumption. The composition of the diet and the caloric values and ultimate disposition of the various foodstuffs were described. Nutritional studies soon led to the discovery of essential components of the diet that were designated "vitamins." So little was known of their mode of action at first that Szent-Györgyi was led to define a vitamin as "something which if you do not eat, makes you sick." It was soon recognized, however, that vitamins are incorporated or converted in the body into relatively small molecules that serve as essential cofactors or co-enzymes for enzymes, large protein molecules that catalyze and are responsible for most of the chemical reactions proceeding in the tissues.

The discovery of the function of vitamins and their relationship to enzyme action led biochemistry into a new period, the era of intermediary metabolism and with it enzymology. It was during this phase that the myriad of chemical interconversions carried out in cells were described in minute detail and sorted into metabolic pathways that define all the intermediate steps in the chemical conversion of a given molecule into its final products. These are the studies that generated the multitude of metabolic maps, which describe the routes of the chemical traffic. These maps contain a variety of straight, branched, diverging, converging, parallel, and cyclical pathways. Nearly every step of every pathway has an enzyme to catalyze it. Not even so simple, spontaneous, and rapid a reaction as the combination of carbon dioxide and water to form carbonic acid, or the reverse, is allowed to proceed freely; it is catalyzed by its own enzyme, carbonic anhydrase. Nature has apparently found it advantageous to have almost all the biochemical reactions enzyme-catalyzed, and it is conceivable that the chief advantage of this arrangement is the potentiality for regulation.

Intermediary metabolism can be viewed as the study of the actions of proteins, specifically enzymes, on small molecules. The enormous number of overlapping and interlocking routes that comprise the pathways of intermediary metabolism obviously offer a great potential for chaos unless rigorously regulated. Regulatory biochemistry is concerned with the controls and regulatory mechanisms that ensure an orderly, coordinated traffic through these routes. There must also be control mechanisms to modify the traffic and adjust it to the changing needs that the cell experiences in response to a variety of physiological situations or stresses, such as changes in functional activity, exposure to hormones and drugs, growth and maturation, altered nutritional states, disease, etc. Since almost all metabolic reactions are catalyzed by enzymes, it is not surprising that their regulation is accomplished mainly by control of enzyme activity. In contrast to intermediary metabolism in which

the emphasis is on the effects of proteins on small molecules, regulatory biochemistry is concerned largely with the effects, both direct and indirect, of small molecules on proteins and, also, of proteins on other proteins. It is for this reason that consideration of the behavior of proteins and the control of enzyme activity permeates the presentations on this topic.

Studies in systems far simpler than nervous tissues have defined some fundamental mechanisms of the control of enzyme activity that must certainly obtain in neural tissues as well. One obvious mechanism is the regulation of the amount of enzyme in the cell, since the rates of enzyme-catalyzed reactions are generally proportional to the concentration of enzyme. It is a little more than a decade ago that the Jacob-Monod model was proposed to explain the induction of the synthesis of specific enzymes by certain small molecules in bacterial cultures in the log phase of growth. This model deservedly had a tremendous impact in biochemistry, but it was at first too quickly and sometimes uncritically applied to explain almost all changes in enzyme activities that occur in mammalian tissues in a variety of conditions. It soon became apparent, however, that stable populations of mammalian cells, constantly turning over their constituents, are not exactly like bacteria multiplying exponentially and that enzyme levels in cells are determined not only by the synthesis of the enzymes but by the balance between their rates of synthesis and degradation. Control of enzyme levels can, therefore, be achieved by regulation of the rate of protein synthesis or the rate of protein degradation.

Enzyme activity can also be regulated by modification of the catalytic efficiency of already existing enzyme molecules. Enzymes are large molecules with very complex three-dimensional structures. Many enzymes exist in aggregates of identical or nonidentical subunits. This structure influences not only the binding affinities of the enzyme for its substrates but also the spatial relationship of the substrates on the surface of the enzyme to each other and to the active catalytic site of the enzyme. The structure of an enzyme is not fixed; it can readily be modified by changes in the conditions of the milieu surrounding it, such as pH, ionic strength, etc. In addition, there are in many enzymes binding sites for specific small molecules, ligands, that may or may not be similar to the substrates of the chemical reaction. These sites and the ligands that they bind are not, however, directly related to the nature and mechanism of the enzyme-catalyzed reaction. They serve only a regulatory function. The binding of the ligand to the regulatory site in the enzyme results in a modification of the three-dimensional structure of the enzyme that is manifested in changes in its kinetic properties. Some enzymes show merely a reversible increase or decrease in activity; others are completely activated or deactivated. This is the essence of allosteric control of enzyme activity. It confers an additional and important mechanism of enzyme regulation, the modification of the catalytic efficiency of existing enzyme molecules without a change in their number.

The organization of this part heavily emphasizes these fundamental mechanisms of biochemical regulation. The first several presentations are directed specifically at the definition, description, and elucidation of these mechanisms, and extensive reference is made to studies in biochemical systems other than neural tissues that serve best to illustrate their mode of operation. That these regulatory mechanisms are also operative in the nervous system is virtually certain; they are unquestionably responsible for many of the biochemical and enzyme changes seen in the brain, especially during postnatal maturation and in response to altered functional activity. Subsequent presentations in the program focus directly on some selected examples of biochemical changes observed in neural tissues that can be examined in the light of the understanding of the basic mechanisms of enzyme regulation provided by the earlier discussions.

71 Principles Underlying the Regulation of Synthesis and Degradation of Proteins in Animal Tissues

ROBERT T. SCHIMKE

ABSTRACT The concentrations of the various protein components of cells, whether they be specific enzymes or components of organelles such as ribosomes or membranes, are the result of a delicate balance between their synthesis and their degradation. Either parameter can be affected by hormonal, nutritional, developmental, and genetic factors. The number of potential sites for regulation of specific protein synthesis, as well as specific protein degradation, are multiple, thereby allowing for multiple regulatory mechanisms that assure a fine control of protein levels as required by a changing environment of the cell and entire organism. This presentation will describe briefly the potential sites for regulation and then describe specific examples of such regulation. To generalize, it can be expected that given the specific organism or cell type or the given developmental, hormonal (etc.), variable, different sites and types of regulatory phenomena will be found.

Insofar as all events in a cell ultimately are directed by the expression of genetic material, it can be stated that gene expression underlies the change in any protein constituent. The question of whether all regulation of protein synthesis in animal cells is directly explicable in terms of the model of the lac repressor is unanswered at the present time. Various types of control can mimic the so-called "transcriptional" model of regulation, i.e., the synthesis or nonsynthesis of specific mRNA, including regulation of the number of genes coding for a given protein (gene amplification), and the regulation of transport of (potential) mRNA from nucleus to cytoplasm. The synthesis of specific mRNA can be controlled by the nature of proteins associated with the chromosome (comparable to the lac repressor protein), or may be specified by unique (specifier) proteins associated with the RNA polymerase (comparable to the sigma factors in prokaryotes).

The rate of protein synthesis (i.e., mRNA translation) is dependent on the number of ribosomes, the concentration of initiation, elongation, and termination factors, as well as aminoacyl-tRNA. In certain instances it can be shown that one or more of these factors is rate limiting. However, the extent to which any of these factors (most specifically, initiation factors and unique isoaccepting tRNAs) is specific for protein synthesis and hence can be a unique and specific regulator, is unknown.

The regulation of protein degradation (turnover) represents an additional means of modulating specific protein contents.

Several general facts concerning this process include: (a) The rate of degradation of a protein is a function of that protein as a substrate for proteolysis. This accounts for the marked heterogeneity of rates of turnover of various proteins. (b) The rate of degradation of a given protein can be markedly altered by ligand interaction, or by mutations in the structure of the protein. (c) The activity of the degradation process can vary. Furthermore, our own data suggest that many, if not all, proteins, either cytoplasmic or those associated with organelles, are degraded as cytoplasmic components and in a monomeric (disassociated) state. The mechanisms for the degradation of proteins are not well understood and need not be uniform for all proteins or for all physiological or developmental states of the cell. Thus, a combination of lysosomal and soluble proteases is likely involved.

The concept to be developed is one in which the protein constituents of a cell are in a continual flux of synthesis and degradation, and of association and disassociation, with multiple controls serving to affect their steady-state levels.

REGULATION OF CELLULAR processes is obviously essential to life. Inasmuch as most significant biochemical reactions depend on catalysis by enzymes, the large measure of control is effected by regulating either the catalytic activity of preexisting enzyme molecules by ligand interaction or covalent modification (see chapter by Daniel Koshland, this volume) or by regulating the content of enzyme molecules, or both. Although the most classical and well-documented examples of enzyme regulation involve microorganisms, most specifically *Escherichia coli*, there is an increasing wealth of examples of adaptation of enzyme levels in animal tissues to a variety of hormonal, pharmacologic, genetic, and physiological variables (see review by Schimke and Doyle, 1970). Such changes do not simply reflect activation and inactivation of enzyme proteins, because agents that inhibit protein synthesis can prevent the increases in enzyme activity. More convincing are studies using combined immunologic and radioisotopic techniques in demonstrating both increased content of immunologically reactive protein and increased isotopically labeled amino acids into specific enzymes.

Central to an understanding of the dynamics of enzyme

ROBERT T. SCHIMKE Department of Pharmacology, Stanford University, Stanford, California regulation in mammalian tissues is the fact that changes in enzyme levels take place against a background of continual synthesis and degradation of proteins, i.e., turnover, as demonstrated so elegantly by Schoenheimer and his co-workers (1942) and studied more recently in other laboratories. Continual degradation of protein may be looked upon as an answer to the problem of how to remove enzymes when they are no longer needed, as part of an adaptive response to an altered metabolic state of a cell. In a rapidly growing bacterium, an unneeded enzyme can be diluted by subsequent cell division. In the generally nongrowing animal cell, intracellular degradation becomes increasingly important for this removal process and hence for controlling enzyme levels. Thus, in terms of understanding mechanisms, control both of synthesis and of degradation of proteins is at the very center of modern molecular biology.

In this presentation, we shall examine some of the underlying properties of the regulation of both protein synthesis and protein degradation, describe certain examples of these processes, and then speculate on mechanisms and approaches to an analysis of mechanisms.

Properties of protein turnover in rat liver

Since regulation of enzyme levels takes place against a background of continual synthesis and degradation, certain properties of this overall process are presented as a basis for subsequent discussions. Although the results presented are limited to rat liver, a number of studies have indicated that these general concepts are applicable to other animal tissues, including the nervous system, as well as *E. coli*.

TURNOVER IS EXTENSIVE Studies of Swick (1958), Buchanan (1961), and Schimke (1964) have indicated that essentially all proteins of rat liver take part in the continual replacement process. These studies have used the general technique of continuous administration of an isotope of known specific activity and subsequent comparison of the specific activity of the isotope isolated from protein with that of the administered isotope. For example, in studies using an algal diet of constant ^{14}C specific activity, Buchanan estimated that approximately 70% of rat liver protein was replaced every 4 to 5 days from the dietary source (Buchanan, 1961). Such replacement cannot represent serum proteins (such as albumin), because the steady state level of such proteins in liver is of the order of only 1 to 2% of total liver protein.

TURNOVER IS LARGELY INTRACELLULAR The life span of hepatic cells is of the order of 160 to 400 days (Buchanan, 1961; MacDonald, 1961; Swick et al., 1956), and hence

the extensive turnover occurring in 4 to 5 days precludes cell replacement as the explanation for the turnover in liver.

THERE IS A MARKED HETEROGENEITY OF RATES OF REPLACEMENT OF DIFFERENT PROTEINS (ENZYMES) Table I provides a representative listing of rates of degradation of various specific proteins and cell organelles of rat liver. More extensive listings of various proteins are given by Schimke and Doyle (1970) and Rechcigl (1971). Remarkable is the wide range of half-lives for these specific proteins, ranging from 11 min for ornithine decarboxylase to 16 days for LDH$_5$. In addition, there is no necessary relationship between half-lives and metabolic functions of the enzymes. For instance glucokinase and LDH$_5$, both involved in carbohydrate metabolism, have markedly different half-lives (30 hr versus 16 days), as do tyrosine aminotransferase and arginase (1.5 hr versus 4 to 5 days), both involved in amino acid catabolism. Perhaps more striking is the lack of correlation between the cell fraction or organelles and the rate of turnover of specific proteins. For instance, δ-aminolevulinate synthetase, a mitochondrial enzyme, has a half-life of 1 hr, whereas the overall (or mean) rate of turnover of mitochondrial proteins is 4 to 5 days. Of particular interest is the relatively rapid turnover of cellular membranes of rat liver (half-lives of 2 to 3 days for endoplasmic reticulum and plasma membranes). Yet for specific enzymes of the endoplasmic reticulum, there is again a remarkable heterogeneity of turnover rates, varying from 2 hr for hydroxymethyl glutaryl CoA reductase to 16 days for NAD glycohydrolase.

This marked heterogeneity has several important implications. (a) Organelles are not turning over as units. Rather the various constituents of organelles, including mitochondria, intracellular membranes, as well as ribosomes (Dice and Schimke, 1972) and plasma membranes (Arias et al., 1969) are being replaced at markedly different rates. This has led us to propose, in addition to the metabolic flux involved in synthesis and degradation, an even less perceptible flux involving the continual association and dissociation of the various macromolecular constituents of cells, including multimeric proteins, complexes of proteins with phospholipids (membranes), and complexes of proteins with nucleic acids (ribosomes and chromatin) (see below). (b) The heterogeneity of turnover rates of different proteins is important for the reflection of altered rates of synthesis and degradation of proteins. As discussed extensively by Berlin and Schimke (1965), the time course of a change in an enzyme level is dependent on the rate of degradation of the protein. Thus only those proteins with short half-lives will change rapidly in content after an altered rate either of synthesis

TABLE I

Half-lives of specific enzymes and subcellular fractions of rat liver

Enzymes	Half-Life	Reference
Ornithine decarboxylase (soluble)	11 min	Russell and Snyder, 1968
δ-Aminolevulinate synthetase (mitochondria)	70 min	Marver et al., 1966
Alanine-aminotransferase (soluble)	0.7–1.0 day	Swick et al., 1968
Catalase (peroxisomal)	1.4 day	Price et al., 1962
Tyrosine aminotransferase (soluble)	1.5 hr	Kenney, 1967
Tryptophan oxygenase (soluble)	2 hr	Schimke et al., 1965
Glucokinase (soluble)	1.25 day	Niemeyer, 1966
Arginase (soluble)	4–5 day	Schimke, 1964
Glutamic-alanine transaminase	2–3 day	Segal and Kim, 1963
Lactate dehydrogenase isozyme-5	16 day	Fritz et al., 1969
Cytochrome c reductase (endoplasmic reticulum)	60–80 hr	Kuriyama et al., 1969
Cytochrome b_5 (endoplasmic reticulum)	100–200 hr	Kuriyama et al., 1969
NAD glycohydrolase (endoplasmic reticulum)	16 day	Bock et al., 1971
Hydroxymethylglutaryl CoA reductase (endoplasmic reticulum)	2–3 hr	Higgins et al., 1971
Acetyl CoA carboxylase (soluble)	2 day	Majerus and Kilburn, 1969
Cell fractions		
Nuclear	5.1 day	Arias et al., 1969
Supernatant	5.1 day	Arias et al., 1969
Endoplasmic reticulum	2.1 day	Arias et al., 1969
Plasma membrane	2.1 day	Arias et al., 1969
Ribosomes	5.0 day	Arias et al., 1969
Mitochondria	4–5 day	Swick et al., 1968

or of degradation. We might propose that for those metabolic pathways in which an alteration in enzyme content regulates the pathway (as opposed to an alteration in catalytic activity of the preexisting protein enzyme), the enzyme in question will have a rapid rate of steady-state turnover.

THERE IS A CORRELATION BETWEEN THE RATE OF DEGRADATION OF PROTEINS IN VITRO AND THEIR RATE OF PROTEOLYTIC ATTACK   This is shown in Figure 1. In such an experiment a double-label technique has been used in which one form of an isotopic amino acid, ^{14}C-leucine, was administered as a single intraperitoneal injection 5 days prior to the administration of ^{3}H-leucine. The animal was killed 6 hr later. The ^{14}C radioactivity then represents those proteins labeled 5 days prior to those labeled with the ^{3}H-leucine. As described by Arias et al. (1969) and employed extensively by Dehlinger and Schimke (1970) and Dice and Schimke (1972), if all proteins are turning over at the same rate, all proteins will have the same ^{3}H/^{14}C ratios, whereas if there is a heterogeneity of rates of turnover of different proteins, those ratios will differ. Proteins with high rates of turnover will have high ^{3}H/^{14}C ratios. The reader is referred to the above papers for a discussion of this technique, to the legend of Figure 1 for details, and to Figure 2 for the use of this technique in another context.

Figure 1 demonstrates that, during proteolysis of 100,000 g supernatant proteins by pronase, the radioactivity that is initially released to a trichloroacetic acid soluble form, i.e., amino acids and small peptides, has high ^{3}H/^{14}C ratios. This result indicates that a nonspecific protease preferentially degrades those proteins with a high rate of turnover in vivo. That this specificity resides with the structure of the proteins is shown by the control experiment in which the proteins were first denatured by 8 M urea at pH 9.5 with subsequent blocking of the sulfhydryl groups followed by proteolysis under conditions of protein and pronase concentrations similar to those employed for the "native" cytoplasmic proteins. After such denaturation proteolysis was more rapid, in keeping with the concept that unfolded, or denatured proteins are better substrates for proteolysis (Linderstrom-Lang, 1950). More importantly, there was now no discrimination between proteins on the basis of their rate of degradation in vivo, i.e., the solubilized radioactivity did not vary in the ^{3}H/^{14}C ratio. This experiment strongly supports the concept that inherent susceptibility of the protein to proteolytic attack is an important factor in establishing the heterogeneity of turnover rates of different proteins.

THERE IS AN APPARENT CORRELATION BETWEEN THE SIZE OF PROTEINS AND THEIR RELATIVE RATES OF DEGRADATION   During the course of studies on the heterogeneity of turnover of proteins of plasma membrane and endoplasmic

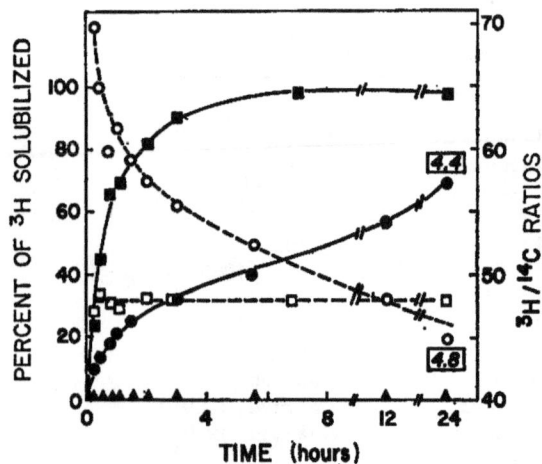

FIGURE 1 Susceptibility of double-labeled supernatant proteins of rat liver to proteolysis by pronase. A rat weighing 120 gm was given 200 μc of ^{14}C-leucine (uniformly labeled, specific activity 300 mc/mM) intraperitoneally, followed 5 days later with 400 μc of ^{3}H-L-leucine (3000 μc/mM). The animal was killed 6 hr later, and following homogenization in 0.25 M sucrose (2.5:1, sucrose to wet weight liver), and initial centrifugation at 1000 and 10,000 × g for 30 min each, a 100,000 × g supernatant fraction was obtained. This fraction was freed of amino acids by passage through a column of Sephadex G-25 equilibrated with 0.05 M potassium phosphate, pH 7.5. To a fraction of the supernatant, urea was added to a final molarity of 8.0, and adjusted to a pH of 9.5 with 3.0 M Tris-OH. After standing at room temperature for 60 min, the sulfhydryl groups were blocked by aminoethylation as described by Cole (1967). The denatured protein was dialyzed overnight against a large excess of 2.0 M urea in 0.05 M potassium phosphate, pH 7.5. The concentration of both the native and denatured proteins was adjusted to 15 mg/ml, and pronase was added to a final concentration of 80 μg/ml. Two ml samples were incubated at 37° with and without pronase, and at the times indicated 100 μl aliquots were removed and added to 0.05 ml of 10% trichloroacetic acid. The precipitates were allowed to sediment at 4° overnight, centrifuged, and 0.25 ml samples removed and extracted 3 times with 2 ml of ethyl ether. Then 0.20 ml samples were counted in a standard dioxane scintillation mixture in the presence of 0.5 ml of NCS solubilizer (Sanno et al., 1970). Samples of proteins were solubilized in 0.5 ml of NCS solubilizer and counted in the same manner. ▲, no pronase; ●, native proteins, cpm; ○, native proteins ^{3}H/^{14}C; ■, denatured proteins cpm; □, denatured proteins ^{3}H/^{14}C.

reticulum, Dehlinger and Schimke (1971) made the observation that relative rates of turnover of proteins, as measured by the double isotope method of Arias et al. (1969) are related to the size of the protein (sub-unit) as electrophoresed on SDS acrylamide gels. Figure 2 depicts this general phenomenon for the proteins of the soluble fraction as fractionated on Sephadex G-200 columns. This correlation was found whether proteins were fractionated as multimeric proteins in the absence of SDS (Figure 2B), or in its presence (Figure 2A). More recently

Dice and Schimke have found this same correlation for proteins of rat liver ribosomes (1972), as well as "soluble" proteins from kidney, brain, and testis (Dice and Schimke, to be published). Such studies have led us to propose that the correlation of size and rate of degradation is based on the overall greater chance of a larger protein being "hit" by an endopeptidase, producing an initial rate-limiting peptide bond cleavage. Since the relative rate of degradation is of the same range of magnitude for the dissociated subunits as for the multimeric proteins (i.e., ^{3}H/^{14}C ratios are similar in Figures 2A and 2B), it is further suggested (Dice et al., in preparation) that proteins were degraded in a dissociated state. This suggestion was also made to explain the fact that this correlation exists for proteins of organelles (ribosomes and membranes), as well as so-called "soluble" proteins. Such studies then suggest another type of dynamic flux of intracellular proteins and organelles, one involving a continual association and dissociation of multimeric proteins and intracellular organelles. Such a concept is consistent with studies on exchange of phospholipids of membranes (Wirtz and Zilversmit, 1968), exchange of ribosomal proteins (Dice and Schimke, 1972; Warner, 1971), and with known association-dissociation phenomena of purified proteins.

Independent regulation of the rates of synthesis and degradation of specific enzymes

There is a wealth of examples of a variety of hormonal, genetic, pharmacologic, and nutritional alterations affecting independently the rates of synthesis and degradation of individual proteins. A number of such examples have been reviewed recently by Schimke and Doyle (1970). Below are presented two such examples, which demonstrate the importance of both synthesis and degradation in controlling specific protein levels.

HORMONE AND SUBSTRATE REGULATION OF TRYPTOPHAN OXYGENASE (PYRROLASE) As shown originally by Knox and Mehler (1951), and studied extensively by Knox and his collaborators (1967) as well as by Feigelson and Greengard (1962), the activity of tryptophan oxygenase can be increased by the administration of either hydrocortisone and other glucocorticoids, or by tryptophan, or certain tryptophan analogues.

Figure 3 shows the time course of increase in tryptophan oxygenase following the administrations of tryptophan, hydrocortisone, or both, to adrenalectomized rats at 4-hour intervals (Schimke et al., 1965). Hydrocortisone resulted in an initial rapid accumulation of enzyme, followed by a plateau after about 8 hr. Tryptophan resulted in a nearly linear increase in enzyme amounting

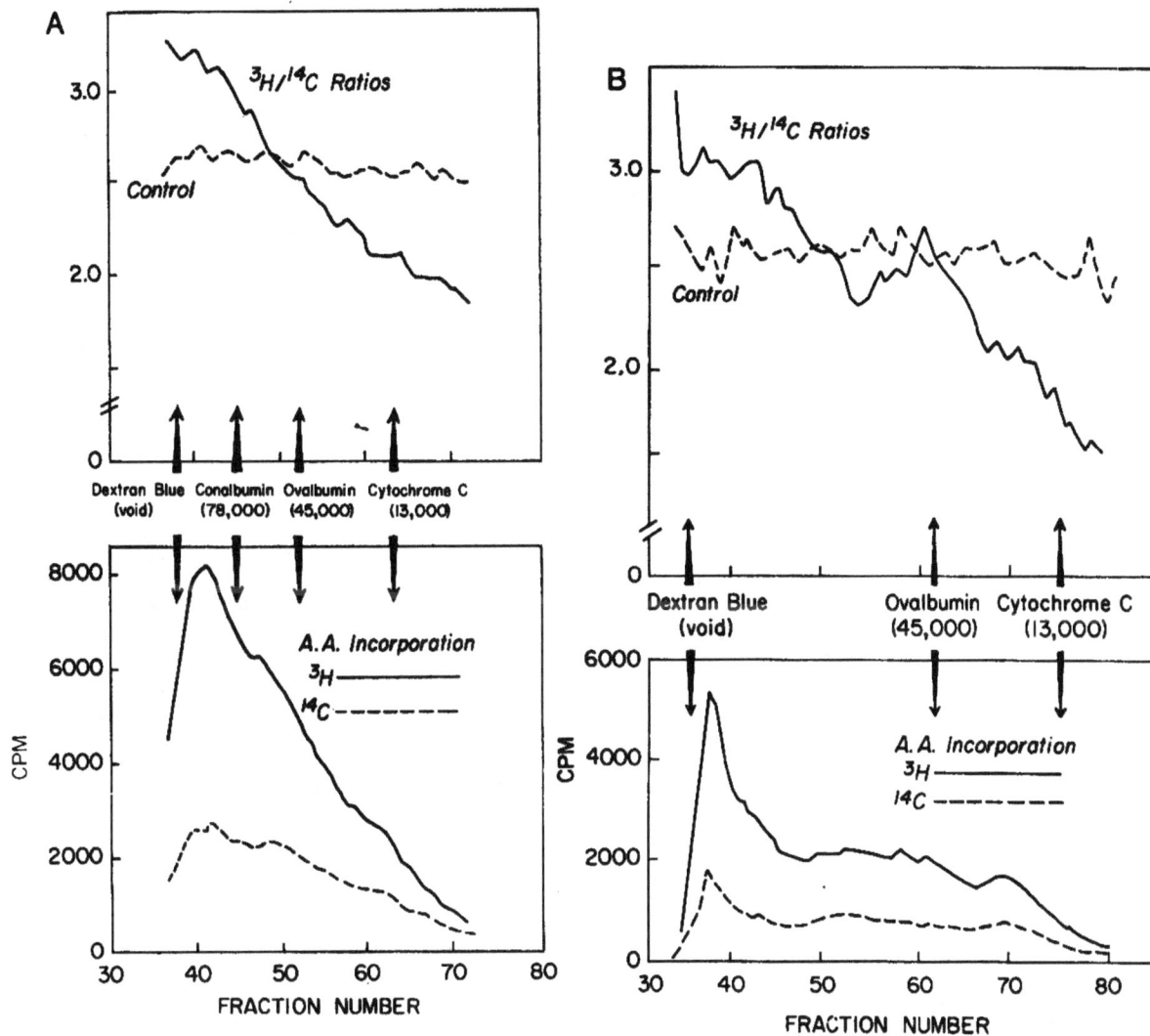

FIGURE 2   Relative rate of degradation of "soluble" proteins of rat liver as a function of molecular size. Relative rates of degradation were estimated by the double isotope method of Arias et al. (1969) in which ^{14}C-leucine is administered to rats four days prior to ^{3}H-leucine administration, with death of animals 4 hr later. The "control" indicates rats receiving both isotope forms of leucine at the same time. High ^{3}H/^{14}C ratio indicates relatively high rates of degradation. Proteins in absence (A) and presence (B) of SDS to disrupt multimeric proteins, were chromatographed on Sephadex G-200 columns. Details are given in Dehlinger and Schimke (1970).

to a 5-fold increase in 16 hr. The administration of both hydrocortisone and tryptophan caused a nearly linear increase of levels 25- to 50-fold greater than basal levels. These time courses of accumulation could be explained on the basis of the theoretical formulation described previously if hydrocortisone increased the rate of enzyme synthesis about 4- to 6-fold without affecting the rate of enzyme degradation, and if tryptophan administration did not appreciably alter the rate of enzyme synthesis but diminished the rate at which the enzyme was inactivated or degraded.

In order to substantiate the conclusions derived from the time course results, experiments were undertaken to study the incorporation and loss of isotopic amino acids from tryptophan oxygenase. In order to assess the effect of hydrocortisone and tryptophan on the rate of enzyme synthesis, studies were undertaken on the short-term incorporation of L-leucine-^{14}C into tryptophan oxygenase. Hydrocortisone or tryptophan, or both, were administered to rats for varying time periods, followed by leucine-^{14}C. Extracts of livers were prepared 40 min after isotope administrations, and the enzyme was isolated by means of the antibody that specifically precipitates tryptophan oxygenase. These results are summarized in Table II. With no treatment, a total of about 1400 cpm were incorporated into tryptophan

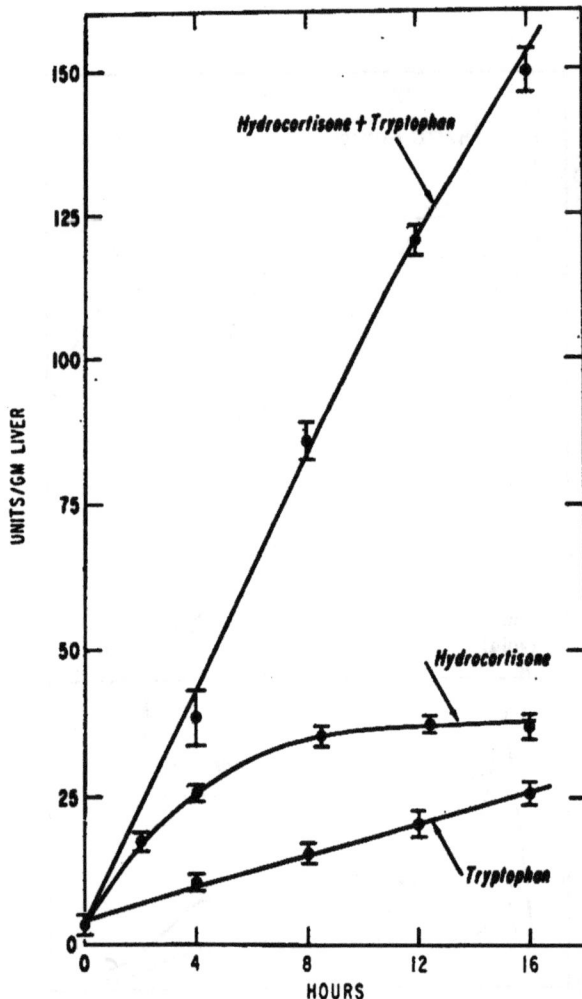

FIGURE 3 The time course of increases in tryptophan oxygenase produced by repeated administrations of hydrocortisone and tryptophan. Adrenalectomized rats weighing 150 to 170 gm each were given injections as follows every 4 hr: 150 mg of L-tryptophan in 12 ml of 0.85% NaCl intraperitoneally and 5 mg of hydrocortisone 21-phosphate subcutaneously. Every 4 hr, the livers of four animals were assayed for tryptophan pyrrolase activity. Brackets indicate ±2 standard errors of the mean (Schimke et al., 1965).

TABLE II
*Forty-minute incorporation of leucine-^{14}C into rat liver
tryptophan oxygenase**

Treatment	Enzyme Activity (units/ gm liver)	Leucine-[14]C Incorporation	
		Tryptophan Oxygenase (total cpm)	Supernatant Protein (cpm/mg)
None	4.2	1368	1190
Hydrocortisone			
4 hr	13.6	5640	1320
12 hr	31.4	6502	1491
Tryptophan			
4 hr	8.2	1620	1564
12 hr	14.1	1670	1165
Hydrocortisone + tryptophan			
4 hr	28.3	7680	1491
12 hr	72.0	7280	1018

*Rats were given repeated doses of hydrocortisone or L-tryptophan, or both, at 4-hr intervals for the times indicated. Each rat was given, 40 min before death, a single intraperitoneal injection of 20 μc of leucine-^{14}C in 1.0 ml of 0.85% NaCl. Results of L-leucine-^{14}C incorporation into tryptophan oxygenase are reported as total net counts per minute in the precipitate from the total DEAE-cellulose extract of two rats. See Schimke et al. (1965) for details.

pyrrolase of livers of two animals during a 40-min period. When hydrocortisone has been administered 4 hr previously, total incorporation into tryptophan oxygenase increased some 4-fold (5640 cpm). After repeated doses of hydrocortisone at 4-hr intervals for 12 hr, the extent of incorporation during a 40-min period remained about 4-fold greater than with no treatment. Tryptophan administration, in contrast, increased only slightly the incorporation (1620 cpm versus 1400 cpm). Hydrocortisone plus tryptophan increased the incorporation in untreated animals about 5-fold. These changes in amount of isotope incorporation into tryptophan oxygenase are to be contrasted with the lack of comparable effects with

total protein. The contrast indicates a high degree of specificity to the hydrocortisone effect. The results, then, indicate that hydrocortisone increased the rate of synthesis of tryptophan oxygenase about 4- to 5-fold.

Evidence that tryptophan prevents the breakdown of the active, immunologically reactive enzyme is shown in Figure 4. In this experiment the enzyme was prelabeled by the administration of leucine-[14]C 60 min before the time indicated as zero. We have found that within 40 min after the administration of a single dose of leucine-^{14}C, incorporation of radioactivity into total liver protein is essentially complete. Therefore any protein synthesized after this time will be derived from unlabeled amino acids. As shown in this experiment, in control animals the amount of enzyme activity and radioactivity present in total protein remained essentially constant over a 9-hr period. However, the radioactivity present in prelabeled enzyme decreased progressively. This, then, is further evidence that there is a continual degradation of the enzyme under basal conditions. When tryptophan was administered, on the other hand, the total amounts of enzyme increased. In contrast to control animals, there was no decrease in the amount of prelabeled enzyme. Thus the substrate, tryptophan, resulted in accumulation of enzyme in large part by preventing degradation of the enzyme in the presence of continued synthesis.

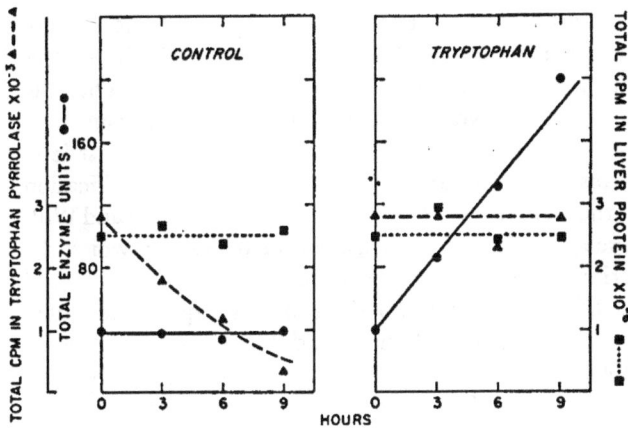

FIGURE 4 Effect of L-tryptophan administration on the loss of tryptophan oxygenase (pyrrolase) prelabeled with L-leucine-^{14}C. Rats were given single injections of 20 μc of L-leucine-^{14}C. Sixty minutes later, two animals were killed. The remainder were given 10 ml of 0.85% NaCl or 10 ml of 0.85% NaCl containing 150 mg of L-tryptophan. These injections were repeated in the remaining animals after 4 and 8 hr. At the times specified, the livers of two animals in each group were removed and frozen immediately. At the end of the experiment, extracts of the livers were prepared, and the radioactivity that was incorporated into tryptophan oxygenase and protein was determined. The values given are for totals of combined extracts of two animals; (●——●) enzyme activity; (▲--▲) total radioactivity in protein precipitated by the tryptophan oxygenase antiserum; (■--■) radioactivity in total cellular protein (Schimke et al., 1965).

REGULATION OF LDH$_5$ ISOZYME LEVELS IN VARIOUS TISSUES OF THE RAT In many instances there are remarkable differences in the specific activities of enzymes catalyzing the same reaction in different tissues. In certain cases, particularly in comparing liver with tissues such as muscle or kidney, this is based on the fact that they represent completely different proteins with different regulatory properties, for example the hexokinase isozymes, including the liver-specific glucokinase (Niemeyer, 1966), and the pyruvate kinase isozymes (Tanaka et al., 1967). One particularly important study is that of Fritz et al. (1969) who have determined the rates of synthesis and degradation of lactate dehydrogenase isozyme-5 in rat liver, heart muscle, and skeletal muscle as summarized in Table III. These workers have found that the tissue differences in enzyme levels were not related solely to rates of synthesis, but that the rate of LDH$_5$ degradation was also markedly different in the different tissues. Thus the half-lives of this isozyme were 16, 1.6, and 31 days in liver, heart muscle, and skeletal muscle, respectively, compared to mean half-lives of 2.2, 1.0, and 22 days for total soluble protein in these same tissues. Thus the same isozyme in different tissues may be degraded at markedly different rates. Hence we cannot assume that differences

TABLE III

Steady-state levels of LDH$_5$ and rates of synthesis and degradation*

Tissue	Enzyme Level (pN/g tissue)	K_s (pM/g/ day)	K_d (day^{-1})	Half-Life†	
Heart	5.5	2.2	0.400	1.6	(1.0)
Muscle	294	65.2	0.018	31	(22.0)
Liver	1600	65.0	0.040	16	(2.2)

*From Fritz et al. (1969).
†Parenthesis indicate values for total soluble protein.

in enzyme levels from tissue to tissue result from differences in rates of synthesis.

The pattern that emerges from these studies, as well as a vast number not discussed, is one of a continual change, in which the rate at which the steady-state complement of specific molecules of a particular enzyme is replaced varies from several hours to many days. In fact, the concept of a "steady state" is most likely a misnomer, and rates of synthesis and degradation of proteins are most likely continually changing in response to dietary, hormonal, and physiologic variables. Thus the constancy of ordered structure and function of cells takes place against a continual flux in the constituent macromolecules, and in fact, change is the only constant.

On the regulation of enzyme synthesis

Figure 5 gives a schematic depiction of the various steps involved in the initial transcription of RNA and DNA, its transport out of the nucleus, its association with ribosomal subunits, release of the completed peptide chain, and finally the assembly of the protein subunits into their functional state, associated with other subunits (enzymes), nucleic acids (ribosomes and chromatin), or phospholipids (membranes). The question of what regulates the final appearance of a protein as an active enzyme or structural unit need not, and in all likelihood does not, have a unique or universal answer. Potentially any of the processes listed, or any single reactant, may be rate limiting.

The most obvious question is whether, as in bacteria, control of protein synthesis is exerted at the level of immediate and continued synthesis of specific mRNA as directed by the interaction of regulatory proteins with a specific region of DNA (Epstein and Beckwith, 1968). There is, indeed, considerable evidence that alterations of RNA metabolism are involved in enzyme regulation in animal tissues. Thus a majority of hormonal, drug, and nutritionally induced increases in enzymes are prevented by the administration of actinomycin D or other inhibitors

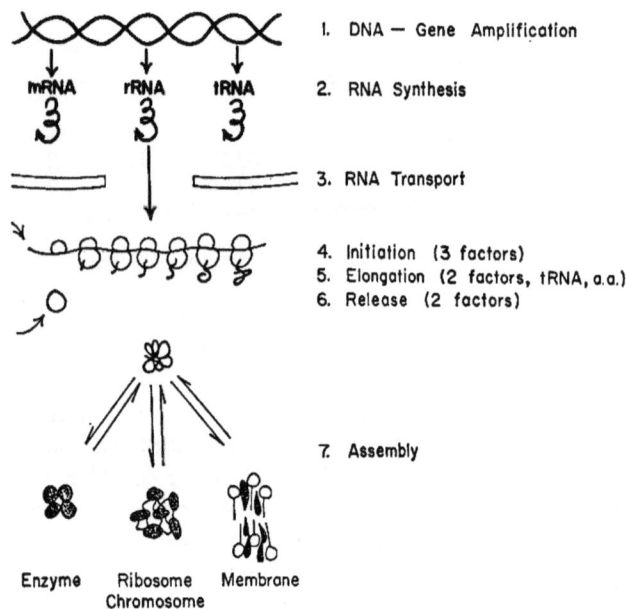

1. DNA — Gene Amplification

2. RNA Synthesis

3. RNA Transport

4. Initiation (3 factors)
5. Elongation (2 factors, tRNA, a.a.)
6. Release (2 factors)

7. Assembly

Enzyme   Ribosome   Membrane
          Chromosome

FIGURE 5 Schematic representation of steps in protein synthesis and possible sites of regulation.

of RNA synthesis. Administration of an inhibitor of RNA synthesis at the time of drug or hormone administration characteristically prevents the increase, whereas delayed administration does not prevent enzyme accumulation (Garren et al., 1964; Greengard and Dewey, 1968). This observation suggests that RNA synthesis is necessary for the initiation of increased synthesis of specific protein, but once that RNA synthesis is accomplished, its utilization can take place for some time. This general finding is in keeping with the concept that mRNAs of animal tissues are relatively long-lived (Pitot et al., 1965; Revel and Hiatt, 1964) when compared to the average 2 or 3 min half-life of bacterial mRNAs (Leive, 1965; Morse et al., 1969). In addition there is ample evidence that some mRNAs, in particular those coding for specific differentiated proteins, are long-lived (Kafatos and Reich, 1968; Palmiter et al., 1971; Papaconstantinou, 1967; Pitot et al., 1965; Wessells and Wilt, 1965; Yaffe and Feldman, 1964). It is the finding of relatively long lives of mRNA that has led to a variety of proposals that regulation can occur at one or more of the many steps that occur subsequent to mRNA synthesis.

It has been customary in studies with animal tissues to differentiate between "transcription" and "translation" as the level at which control of specific protein synthesis is exerted. Operationally this distinction has been based

primarily on whether actinomycin D prevents the increase in enzyme content. The use of actinomycin D for this distinction is unsound for a variety of reasons. Thus the use of actinomycin D cannot distinguish between an effect on the synthesis or nonsynthesis of mRNA (the strictly transcriptional model), one in which gene amplification is the primary effect (Arias et al., 1969; Aronson and Wilt, 1969; Dawid and Brown, 1968) or the case in which the primary effect is on mRNA transport, where potential mRNA may be synthesized but is rapidly degraded within the nucleus (Aronson and Wilt, 1969; Attardi et al., 1966; Harris, 1968; Scherrer et al., 1966; Shearer and McCarthy, 1967; Soeiro et al., 1968), unless it is transported into the cytoplasm and there utilized for protein synthesis. Georgiev (1967) has reviewed evidence suggesting that actinomycin D may inhibit the transport phenomenon. In addition, when using actinomycin D, it is never clear that the inhibition of the specific mRNA for the enzyme in question is the event that prevents enzyme accumulation. Thus the inhibition of synthesis of a labile RNA species necessary for the utilization of a specific mRNA may be the underlying action of actinomycin D in a given case.

In addition to gene amplification, altered rates of synthesis of mRNA, and transport of mRNA into the cytoplasm at sites at which regulation can take place, various steps in the utilization of mRNA have been proposed for regulation. Thus Heywood (1970) has suggested that there is specificity for the initiation of myosin mRNA as studied in the reticulocyte protein synthesizing system. Regulation of the stability of mRNA species has been championed in the so-called *membron* theory of Pitot et al. (1969). Tomkins et al. (1969) have developed a theory of a cytoplasmic repressor protein that binds to mRNA, preventing its translation, and at the same time initiating its degradation. Regulation of ribosome function on the basis of variations in tRNA acceptor properties (Kano-Sueoka and Sueoka, 1966; Maenpaa and Bernfield, 1970), or by the synthesis of specific proteins as studied by Martin and Wool (1968), or as controlled by phosphorylation of ribosomal proteins (Kabat, 1971) have been proposed as regulatory sites. Amino acid availability will obviously regulate the rate of protein synthesis. Potter et al. (1968) have described the influx and efflux of amino acids from rat liver as a function of feeding schedules. Hence, in the intact animal, the supply of amino acids in the liver is not constant. The cyclic variations in tyrosine transaminase activity (Wurtman and Axelrod, 1967) and the effect of growth hormone on tyrosine transaminase (Kenney and Albritton, 1965; Labrie and Korner, 1968a) may be explained on the basis of amino acid availability, altering rates of synthesis of a rapidly degraded enzyme. Munro (1968) and Sidransky et al. (1968) have shown that the profile of rat liver polysomes is extremely sensitive to amino acid availability, and in particular to the availability of tryptophan. This finding may underlie the effect of low doses of tryptophan in increasing activity of serine dehydratase (Peraino et al., 1965), tyrosine transaminase (Labrie and Korner, 1968a), and tryptophan pyrrolase (Labrie and Korner, 1968a). Last, control of protein synthesis at the level of release of specific peptides has been suggested (Cline and Bock, 1966).

Clearly what is needed is the ability to isolate all potential reactants in the chain of specific protein synthesis, including specific polysomes with their (specific or nonspecific) initiation and release factors, specific mRNA, and genes. Recent advances in the ability to utilize mammalian mRNAs for protein synthesis, including globin chains (Gurdon et al., 1971; Lockard and Lingrel, 1969), light immunoglobulin chains (Stavnezer and Huang, 1971), and ovalbumin (Rhoads et al., 1973), and the development of methodology for isolation of specific polysomes utilizing immunoprecipitation techniques (Allen and Terrence, 1968; Holme et al., 1971; Schubert, 1968; Takagi and Ogata, 1971), should allow for more searching analyses of the question of what is rate limiting.

The isolation and quantification of specific mRNAs should then allow for a more profound analysis of the nature of the RNA that turns over rapidly in the nucleus (Aronson and Wilt, 1969; Attardi et al., 1966; Harris, 1968; Scherrer et al., 1966; Soeiro et al., 1968), and perhaps a better understanding of reiterated DNA sequences of animal tissue (Britten and Kohne, 1968; McCarthy and McConaughy, 1968) than is currently available from the multitude of hybridization studies using DNA and so-called mRNAs of unknown properties. Obviously the eventual goal will be an understanding of interactions of proteins and DNA in the regulation of gene expression, including the role of various nuclear and chromosomal protein fractions (histones and acidic proteins), and enzymatic modifications of these proteins by phosphorylation, acetylation, and so on (Stellwagen and Cole, 1969).

Enzyme degradation

Any understanding of the molecular mechanisms for degradation of proteins (enzymes) must take into account certain fundamental properties of such turnover as follows:

1. The degradation appears to be random, inasmuch as the loss of labeled protein during chase period, or fall of enzyme activity following elevation to a high level, follows first-order kinetics.

2. There is a marked heterogeneity of turnover rates of individual proteins.

3. The rate constant of degradation is in many cases characteristic of a given protein but in other cases can be markedly altered.

4. There is a general correlation between the size of a protein and its relative rate of degradation.

Two general mechanisms can be considered, as summarized in Figure 6.

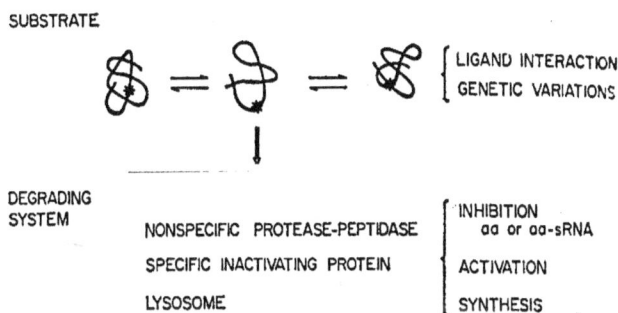

FIGURE 6 Summary of possible means of regulating protein degradation.

PROPERTIES OF THE PROTEIN MOLECULE AS A SUBSTRATE FOR DEGRADATION Protein molecules can exist in a number of different conformational states of varying degrees of detection. A protein molecule might be subject to degradation only when it assumes certain conformations. Thus a heterogeneity of degradation rates could exist, depending on the number and nature of particularly labile peptide bonds exposed in certain conformations. In addition, the interactions of proteins with various ligands, including other proteins, lipids, and small molecules, can alter such conformations and thereby alter proteins as substrates for inactivation. The model that emerges, then, is one in which protein molecules are individually available to a degradative process that is present at all times. Shifting concentrations of substrates, cofactors, and so on, as occur under various hormonal and physiological conditions, would lead to a variety of effects on specific enzymes, either to stabilize or labilize them. Such a concept has also been expressed by Grisolia (1964) and Pine (1966, 1967). Consistent with this is the finding that there is a general correlation between known rates of degradation of proteins in vivo and their rate of inactivation by trypsin and chymotrypsin (Bond, 1971). In addition, Goldberg (1972) has recently shown that when amino acid analogs are incorporated into the proteins in E. coli, protein degradation is accelerated, either as studied in vivo or in extracts. In addition, the effects of ligands to alter heat and proteolytic inactivation of numerous proteins are well known (Green and Neurath, 1954).

Such a concept could also explain the development of heterogeneity of rate constants of degradation. Taking a cue from mutations in *E. coli*, which decrease the stability of the lac repressor (Platt et al., 1970), and an arginine tRNA synthetase (Williams and Neidhardt, 1969), as well as the mutations that affect the stability of catalase (Matsubara et al., 1967) and glucose-6-phosphate dehydrogenase (Yoshida et al., 1967), we can readily envisage the retention of those mutations that either increase or decrease stability of a protein, depending on whether rapid or slow turnover is advantageous to the organism.

The correlation between the size of a protein and its relative rate of degradation does not hold for specific proteins, such as LDH_5, arginase, and tyrosine aminotransferase, all of which are of approximately the same molecular size (Auricchio et al., 1970; Castellino and Barker, 1968; Hirsch-Kolb and Greenberg, 1968) but have markedly different half-lives of 16 days (Fritz et al., 1969), 4 to 5 days (Schimke, 1964), and 1.5 hr (Kenney, 1967), respectively. Dehlinger and Schimke (1970) have proposed that the degradation may not occur as the multimeric protein but rather in the dissociated state, a proposal that is in keeping with the suggestion of Fritz et al. (1971). Thus one of the rate limiting parameters for degradation to be considered should be the facility of dissociation of the protein into subunits.

ALTERATIONS IN ACTIVITY OF A DEGRADATIVE PROCESS
In the above model the activity of the degradative process was assumed to be in excess. It is also conceivable that the rate of degradation may be dependent on the activity of the degrading system, as controlled by activation inhibition, translocation within the cell, or de novo synthesis of degrading enzymes. Considerations of enzymatic mechanisms are hampered by lack of suitable mutants in the degradative process itself. Another problem involves the identification of the products of specific protein degradation once a protein has lost enzymatic activity or immunologic reactivity. Several curious observations are of note that should be explained in the formulation of a suitable mechanism(s) for degradation. In both animal and bacterial systems, inhibition of energy production and protein synthesis inhibits protein degradation (see Schimke et al., 1970 for detailed review). Various explanations have been offered for such observations, including cofactor requirements (Penn, 1961), necessity for maintaining structural integrity of organelles such as lysosomes (Brostrom and Jeffay, 1970), and requirement for continued synthesis of degradative enzymes that are turning over rapidly (Kenney, 1967). More indirect, but equally plausible from the experimental data available, are effects of accumulated amino acids, tRNA species, and so on, that may regulate by ligand interaction the activity of degradative enzymes or specific (enzyme) substrates.

One obvious candidate for a degradative system is lysosome, which occurs in virtually all cells (DeDuve and Wattiaux, 1966). Lysosomes are intracellular organelles that contain acid hydrolases and are currently conceived as involved in the autophagy of discrete areas of cytoplasm. It is not difficult to conceive that lysosomes are involved in that protein degradation whose properties involve randomness and heterogeneity of degradation rate constants among different proteins, whether so-called soluble proteins or those associated with membranes or ribosomes. Thus some mechanism would be required for the recognition of whether a protein molecule were to be degraded and perhaps involve transport into a lysosome, acetylation, formylation, or as recently suggested, deamidation (Robinson et al., 1970). It seems reasonable to this author to propose that the system of lysosomes is important where cell involution or gross changes in rates of protein degradation occur, such as starvation and cell death, whereas the degradation that occurs in normal steady-state conditions involves a system(s) not clearly understood at present (Hartley, 1960). This could involve lysosomes, but acting as a sieve, rather than in an "all-or-none" fashion.

Another possibility is that there are specific degrading enzymes for specific proteins. There are examples of proteins or enzymes that appear to inhibit or inactivate specific enzymes (Blobel and Potter, 1966; Bonsignore et al., 1968; Dvorak et al., 1966; Gancedo and Holzer, 1968; Messenguy and Wiame, 1969). In addition, studies by Tata (1966) and by Gross and Lapiere (1962) on degeneration of amphibian tail during thyroxine-induced metamorphosis and of Houck et al. (1968) on the glucocorticoid-induced degeneration of skin of rats suggest that de novo synthesis of specific proteolytic enzymes is required for these instances of tissue involution.

At one extreme, then, we might propose that the degradation of each protein requires a specific protein. This, however, is impossible, because the continual replacement of essentially all proteins would require that there exist a protein to degrade a protein . . . ad infinitum. It is most likely that, just as there are a number of different enzymes that hydrolyze RNA in an organism such as *E. coli*, there are also a number of different types of proteases in animal cells (Hartley, 1960) performing different functional tasks at different sites and times, the sum total of which results in continual protein degradation.

REFERENCES

ALLEN, E. R., and C. F. TERRENCE, 1968. Immunochemical and ultrastructural studies of myosin synthesis. *Proc. Natl. Acad. Sci. USA* 60:1209–1215.

ARIAS, I. M., D. DOYLE, and R. T. SCHIMKE, 1969. Studies on the synthesis and degradation of proteins of the endoplasmic reticulum of rat liver. *J. Biol. Chem.* 244:3303–3315.

ARONSON, A. I., and F. H. WILT, 1969. Properties of nuclear RNA in sea urchin embryos. *Proc. Natl. Acad. Sci. USA* 62:186–193.

ATTARDI, G., H. PARNAS, M-I. H. HWANG, and B. ATTARDI, 1966. Giant-size rapidly labeled nuclear ribonucleic acid and cytoplasmic messenger ribonucleic acid in immature duck erythrocytes. *J. Mol. Biol.* 20:145–182.

AURICCHIO, F., F. VALIEROTE, G. TOMKINS, and W. RILEY. 1970. Studies on the structure of tyrosine aminotransferase. *Biochim. Biophys. Acta* 221:307–313.

BERLIN, C. M., and R. T. SCHIMKE, 1965. Influence of turnover rates on the responses of enzymes to cortisone. *Mol. Pharmacol.* 1:149–156.

BLOBEL, G., and V. R. POTTER, 1966. Relation of ribonuclease and ribonuclease inhibition to the isolation of polysomes from rat liver. *Proc. Natl. Acad. Sci. USA* 55:1283–1288.

BOCK, K. W., P. SIEKEVITZ, and G. E. PALADE, 1971. Localization and turnover studies of membrane nicotinamide adenine dinucleotide glycohydrolase in rat liver. *J. Biol. Chem.* 246:188–195.

BOND, J. S., 1971. A comparison of the proteolytic susceptibility of several rat liver enzymes. *Biochem. Biophys. Res. Commun.* 43:333–339.

BONSIGNORE, A., A. DEFLORA, M. A. MANGIAROTTI, I. LORENZONI, and S. ALEMA, 1968. A new hepatic protein inactivating glucose 6-phosphate dehydrogenase. *Biochem. J.* 106:147–154.

BRITTEN, R. J., and D. W. KOHNE, 1968. Repeated sequences in DNA. *Science* 161:529–540.

BROSTROM, C. O., and H. JEFFAY, 1970. Protein catabolism in rat liver homogenates. A reevaluation of the energy requirement for protein catabolism. *J. Biol. Chem.* 245:4001–4008.

BUCHANAN, D. L., 1961. Total carbon turnover measured by feeding a uniformly labeled diet. *Arch. Biochem. Biophys.* 94:500–511.

CASTELLINO, F. J., and R. BARKER, 1968. Examination of the dissociation of multichain proteins in guanidine hydrochloride by membrane osmometry. *Biochemistry* 7:2207–2217.

CLINE, A. L., and R. M. BOCK, 1966. Translational control of gene expression. *Cold Spring Harbor Symp. Quant. Biol.* 31:321–333.

COLE, D., 1967. δ-Aminoethylation. In *Methods in Enzymology*, Vol. XI, S. P. Colowick and N. O. Kaplan, eds. New York: Academic Press, pp. 315–317.

DAWID, I. B., and D. M. BROWN, 1968. Specific gene amplification in oocytes. *Science* 160:272–280.

DEDUVE, C., and R. WATTIAUX, 1966. Functions of lysosomes. *Ann. Rev. Physiol.* 28:435–492.

DEHLINGER, P. J., and R. T. SCHIMKE, 1970. Effect of size on the relative rate of degradation of rat liver soluble proteins. *Biochem. Biophys. Res. Commun.* 40:1473–1480.

DICE, J. F., and R. T. SCHIMKE, 1972. Turnover and exchange of ribosomal proteins from rat liver. *J. Biol. Chem.* 247:98–111.

DVORAK, H. F., Y. ANRAKU, and L. A. HEPPEL, 1966. The occurrence of a protein inhibitor for 5′-nucleotidase in extracts of *Escherichia coli*. *Biochem. Biophys. Res. Commun.* 24:628–632.

EPSTEIN, W., and J. R. BECKWITH, 1968. Regulation of gene expression. *Ann. Rev. Biochem.* 37:411–436.

FEIGELSON, P., M. FEIGELSON, and O. GREENGARD, 1962. Comparison of the mechanisms of hormonal and substrate induction of rat liver tryptophan pyrrolase. *Recent Progr. Hormone Res.* 18:491–507.

FRITZ, P. J., E. L. WHITE, E. S. VESELL, and K. M. PRUITT, 1969. The roles of synthesis and degradation in determining tissue concentrations of lactate dehydrogenase-5. *Proc. Natl. Acad. Sci. USA* 62:558–565.

FRITZ, P. J., E. L. WHITE, E. S. VESSELL, and K. M. PRUITT, 1971. *Nature New Biol.* 230:119–122.

GANCEDO, C., and H. HOLZER, 1968. Enzymatic inactivation of glutamine synthetase in *Enterobacteriaceae*. *Eur. J. Biochem.* 4:190–192.

GARREN, L. D., R. R. HOWELL, G. M. TOMKINS, and R. M. CROCCO, 1964. A paradoxical effect of actinomycin D: The mechanism of regulation of enzyme synthesis by hydrocortisone. *Proc. Natl. Acad. Sci. USA* 52:1121–1129.

GEORGIEV, G. P., 1967. The nature and biosynthesis of nuclear ribonucleic acids. *Progr. Nucleic Acid. Res. Mol. Biol.* 6:259–351.

GOLDBERG, A. L., 1972. *Nature New Biol.* 240:147–150.

GREEN, N. M., and H. NEURATH, 1954. Proteolytic enzymes. In *The Proteins*, Vol. II, Part B, H. Neurath and K. Bailey, eds. New York: Academic Press, pp. 1057–1198.

GREENGARD, O., and H. K. DEWEY, 1968. The developmental formation of liver glucose 6-phosphatase and reduced nicotinamide adenine dinucleotide phosphate dehydrogenase in fetal rats treated with thyroxine. *J. Biol. Chem.* 243:2745–2749.

GRISOLIA, S., 1964. The catalytic environment and its biological implications. *Physiol. Rev.* 44:657–712.

GROSS, J., and C. M. LAPIERE, 1962. Collagenolytic activity in amphibian tissues: A tissue culture assay. *Proc. Natl. Acad. Sci. USA* 48:1014–1022.

GURDON, J. B., C. D. LANE, H. R. WOODLAND, and G. MARBAIX, 1971. Use of frog eggs and oocytes for the study of messenger RNA and its translation in living cells. *Nature (Lond.)* 233:177–182.

HARRIS, H., 1968. *Nucleus and Cytoplasm*. London: Oxford University Press.

HARTLEY, B. S., 1960. Proteolytic enzymes. *Ann. Rev. Biochem.* 29:45–72.

HEYWOOD, S., 1970. Specificity of mRNA binding factor in eukaryotes. *Proc. Natl. Acad. Sci. USA* 67:1782–1788.

HIGGINS, M., T. KAWACHI, and H. RUDNEY, 1971. The mechanism of the diurnal variation of hepatic HMG-CoA reductase activity in the rat. *Biochem. Biophys. Res. Commun.* 45:138–150.

HIRSCH-KOLB, H., and D. M. GREENBERG, 1968. Molecular characteristics of rat liver arginase. *J. Biol. Chem.* 243:6123–6129.

HOLME, G., S. L. BOYD, and A. H. SEHON, 1971. Precipitation of polyribosomes with pepsin digested antibodies. *Biochem. Biophys. Res. Commun.* 45:240–245.

HOUCK, J. C., V. K. SHARMA, Y. M. PATEL, and J. A. GLADNER, 1968. Induction of collagenolytic and proteolytic activities by anti-inflammatory drugs in the skin and fibroblast. *Biochem. Pharmacol.* 17:2081–2090.

KABAT, D., 1971. Phosphorylation of ribosomal proteins in rabbit reticulocytes. A cell-free system with ribosomal protein kinase activity. *Biochemistry* 10:197–203.

KAFATOS, F. C., and J. REICH, 1968. Stability of differentiation-specific and non-specific messenger RNA in insect cells. *Proc. Natl. Acad. Sci. USA* 60:1458–1465.

KANO-SUEOKA, T., and N. SUEOKA, 1966. Modification of leucyl-sRNA after bacteriophage infection. *J. Mol. Biol.* 20:183–209.

KENNEY, F. T., 1967. Turnover of rat liver tyrosine transaminase: Stabilization after inhibition of protein synthesis. *Science* 156:525–528.

KENNEY, F. T., and W. L. ALBRITTON, 1965. Repression of enzyme synthesis at the translational level and its hormonal control. *Proc. Natl. Acad. Sci. USA* 54:1693–1698.

KNOX, W. E., and A. H. MEHLER, 1951. The adaptive increase of the tryptophan peroxidase-oxidase system of liver. *Science* 113:237–238.

KNOX, W. E., and M. M. PIRAS, 1967. Tryptophan pyrrolase of liver, III. Conjugation in vivo during cofactor induction by tryptophan pyrrolase. *J. Biol. Chem.* 242:2965–2969.

KURIYAMA, T., T. OMURA, P. SIEKEVITZ, and G. E. PALADE, 1969. Effects of phenobarbital on the synthesis and degradation of the protein components of rat liver microsomal membranes. *J. Biol. Chem.* 244:2017–2026.

LABRIE, F., and A. KORNER, 1968a. Actinomycin sensitive induction of tyrosine transaminase and tryptophan pyrrolase by amino acids and tryptophan. *J. Biol. Chem.* 243:1116–1119.

LEIVE, L., 1965. RNA degradation and the assembly of ribosomes in actinomycin-treated *Escherichia coli. J. Mol. Biol.* 13:862–875.

LINDERSTROM-LANG, K., 1950. Structure and enzymatic breakdown of proteins. *Cold Spring Harbor Symp. Quant. Biol.* 14:117–126.

LOCKARD, R. E., and J. B. LINGREL, 1969. The synthesis of mouse hemoglobin β-chains in a rabbit reticulocyte cell-free system programmed with mouse reticulocyte 9S RNA. *Biochem. Biophys. Res. Commun.* 37:204–212.

MACDONALD, R. A., 1961. "Lifespan" of liver cells. *Arch. Intern. Med.* 107:335–343.

MAENPAA, P. H., and M. R. BERNFIELD, 1970. A specific hepatic transfer RNA for phosphoserine. *Proc. Natl. Acad. Sci. USA* 67:688–695.

MAJERUS, P. W., and E. KILBURN, 1969. Acetyl coenzyme A carboxylase. The roles of synthesis and degradation in regulation of enzyme levels in rat liver. *J. Biol. Chem.* 244:6254–6262.

MARTIN, T. E., and I. G. WOOL, 1968. Formation of active hybrids from subunits of muscle ribosomes from normal and diabetic rats. *Proc. Natl. Acad. Sci. USA* 60:569–574.

MARVER, H. S., A. COLLINS, D. P. TSCHUDY, and M. RECHCIGL, JR., 1966. δ-Aminolevulinic acid synthetase. *J. Biol. Chem.* 241:4323–4329.

MATSUBARA, S., H. SUTER, and H. AEBI, 1967. Fractionation of erythrocyte catalase from normal, hypocatalatic and acatalatic humans. *Humangenetik* 4:29–41.

MCCARTHY, B. J., and B. L. MCCONAUGHY, 1968. Related base sequences in the DNA of simple and complex organisms. *Biochem. Genet.* 2:37.

MESSENGUY, F., and J. WIAME, 1969. The control of ornithine-transcarbamylase activity by arginase in *Saccharomyces cerevisiae. FEBS Letter* 3:47–49.

MORSE, D. E., R. MOSTELLER, R. F. BAKER, and C. YANOFSKY, 1969. Direction of in vivo degradation of tryptophan messenger RNA—a correction. *Nature (Lond.)* 223:40–43.

MUNRO, H. N., 1968. Role of amino acid supply in regulating ribosome function. *Fed. Proc.* 27:1231–1237.

NIEMEYER, H., 1966. Regulation of glucose-phosphorylating enzymes. *Natl. Cancer Inst. Monograph* 27:29–40.

PALACIOS, R., R. D. PALMITER, and R. T. SCHIMKE, 1971. Identification and isolation of ovalbumin-synthesizing polysomes. *J. Biol. Chem.* 247:2316–2321.

PALMITER, R. D., T. OKA, and R. T. SCHIMKE, 1971. Modulation of ovalbumin synthesis by estradiol-17β and actinomycin D as studied in explants of chick oviduct in culture. *J. Biol. Chem.* 246:724–737.

PAPACONSTANTINOU, J., 1967. Molecular aspects of lens cell differentiation. *Science* 156:338–346.

PENN, N. W., 1961. Metabolism of the protein molecule in a rat liver mitochondrial fraction. *Biochim. Biophys. Acta* 53:490–494.

PERAINO, C., R. C. BLAKE, and H. C. PITOT, 1965. Studies on the induction and repression of enzymes in rat liver. *J. Biol. Chem.* 240:3039–3043.

PINE, M. J., 1966. Metabolic control of intracellular proteolysis in growing and resting cells of *Escherichia coli. J. Bacteriol.* 93:847–850.

PINE, M. J., 1967. Intracellular protein breakdown in the L1210 ascites leukemia. *Cancer Res.* 27:522–525.

PITOT, H. C., C. PERAINO, C. LAMAR, JR., and A. L. KENNAN, 1965. Template stability of some enzymes in rat liver and hepatoma. *Proc. Natl. Acad. Sci. USA* 54:845–851.

PITOT, H. C., N. SLADEK, W. RAGLAND, R. K. MURRAY, G. MOYER, H. D. SOLING, and J-P. JOST, 1969. A possible role of the endoplasmic reticulum in the regulation of genetic expression: The membron concept. In *Microsomes and Drug Oxidations*, J. R. Gillette, A. H. Conney, G. J. Cosmides, R. W. Estabrook, J. R. Fouts, and G. J. Mannering, eds. New York: Academic Press, p. 59.

PLATT, T., J. H. MILLER, and K. WEBER, 1970. In vivo degradation of mutant lac repressor. *Nature (Lond.)* 228:1154–1156.

POTTER, V. R., E. F. BARIL, M. WATANABE, and E. D. WHITTLE, 1968. Systematic oscillations in metabolic functions in liver from rats adapted to controlled feeding schedules. *Fed. Proc.* 27:1238.

PRICE, V. E., W. R. STERLING, V. A. TARANTOLA, R. W. HARTLEY, JR., and M. RECHCIGL, JR., 1962. The kinetics of catalase synthesis and destruction in vivo. *J. Biol. Chem.* 237:3468–3475.

RECHCIGL, M., JR., 1971. Intracellular protein turnover and the roles of synthesis and degradation in regulation of enzyme levels. In *Enzyme Synthesis and Degradation in Mammalian Systems.* Baltimore: University Park Press, p. 236.

REVEL, M., and H. H. HIATT, 1964. Elovich decay of free radicals in a photosynthetic system as evidence for electron transport across an interfacial activation energy barrier. *Proc. Natl. Acad. Sci. USA* 51:809–818.

RHOADS, R. E., G. S. MCKNIGHT, and R. T. SCHIMKE, 1973. *J. Biol. Chem.* 248:2031–2039.

ROBINSON, A. B., J. H. MCKERROW, and P. CARY, 1970. Controlled deamidation of peptides and proteins: An experimental hazard and a possible biological timer. *Proc. Natl. Acad. Sci. USA* 66:753–757.

RUSSELL, D., and S. H. SNYDER, 1968. Amine synthesis in rapidly growing tissues: Ornithine decarboxylase activity in regenerating rat liver, chick embryo, and various tumors. *Proc. Natl. Acad. Sci. USA* 60:1420–1427.

SANNO, Y., M. HOLZER, and R. T. SCHIMKE, 1970. Studies of a mutation affecting pyrimidine degradation in inbred mouse strains. *J. Biol. Chem.* 245:5668.

SCHERRER, K., L. MARCAUD, F. ZAJDELA, I. M. LONDON, and F. GROS, 1966. Patterns of RNA metabolism in a differentiated cell: A rapidly labeled, unstable 60S RNA with messenger properties in duck erythroblasts. *Proc. Natl. Acad. Sci. USA* 56:1571–1578.

SCHIMKE, R. T., 1964. Enzymes of arginine metabolism in cell culture: Studies on enzyme induction and repression. *Natl. Cancer Inst. Monograph* 13:197–217.

SCHIMKE, R. T., 1964. The importance of both synthesis and degradation in the control of arginase levels in rat liver. *J. Biol. Chem.* 239:3808–3817.

SCHIMKE, R. T., 1970. Regulation of protein degradation in mammalian tissues. In *Mammalian Protein Metabolism*, H. N. Munro, ed. New York: Academic Press, p. 177.

SCHIMKE, R. T., and D. DOYLE, 1970. Control of enzyme levels in animal tissues. *Ann. Rev. Biochem.* 39:929–976.

SCHIMKE, R. T., E. W. SWEENEY, and C. M. BERLIN, 1965. The roles of synthesis and degradation in the control of rat liver tryptophan pyrrolase. *J. Biol. Chem.* 240:322–331.

SCHOENHEIMER, R., 1942. *The Dynamic State of Body Constituents.* Cambridge, Mass.: Harvard University Press.

SCHUBERT, D., 1968. Immunoglobin assembly in a mouse myeloma. *Proc. Natl. Acad. Sci. USA* 60:683–690.

SEGAL, H. L., and Y. S. KIM, 1963. Glucocorticoid stimulation of the biosynthesis of a glutamic-alanine transaminase. *Proc. Natl. Acad. Sci. USA* 50:912–918.

SHEARER, R. W., and B. J. McCARTHY, 1967. Evidence for ribonucleic acid molecules restricted to the cell nucleus. *Biochemistry* 6:283–289.

SIDRANSKY, H., D. S. R. SARMA, M. BONGIORNO, and E. VERNEY, 1968. Effect of dietary tryptophan on hepatic polyribosomes and protein synthesis in fasted mice. *J. Biol. Chem.* 243:1123–1132.

SOEIRO, R., M. H. VAUGHAN, J. R. WARNER, and J. E. DARNELL, JR., 1968. The turnover of nuclear DNA-like RNA in HeLa cells. *J. Cell. Biol.* 39:112–118.

STAVNEZER, J., and R. C. C. HUANG, 1971. Synthesis of a mouse immunoglobulin light chain in a rabbit reticulocyte cell-free system. *Nature New Biol.* 230:172–176.

STELLWAGEN, R. H., and R. D. COLE, 1969. Chromosomal proteins. *Ann. Rev. Biochem.* 38:951–990.

SWICK, R. W., A. L. KOCH, and D. T. HANDA, 1956. The measurement of nucleic acid turnover in rat liver. *Arch. Biochem. Biophys.* 63:226–242.

SWICK, R. W., A. K. REXROTH, and J. L. STANGE, 1968. The metabolism of mitochondrial proteins. III. The dynamic state of rat liver mitochondria. *J. Biol. Chem.* 243:3581–3587.

SWICK, R. W., 1958. Measurement of protein turnover in rat liver. *J. Biol. Chem.* 231:751–764.

TAKAGI, M., and K. OGATA, 1971. Isolation of serum albumin-synthesizing polysomes from rat liver. *Biochem. Biophys. Res. Commun.* 42:125–131.

TANAKA, T., Y. HARANO, F. SUE, and H. MORIMURA, 1967. Crystallization, characterization and metabolic regulation of two types of pyruvate kinase isolated from rat tissues. *J. Biochem. (Tokyo)* 62:71–91.

TATA, J. R., 1966. Requirement for RNA and protein synthesis for induced regression of the tadpole tail in organ culture. *Develop. Biol.* 13:77–94.

TOMKINS, G. M., T. D. GELEHRTER, D. GRANNER, D. MARTIN, JR., H. H. SAMUELS, and E. B. THOMPSON, 1969. Control of specific gene expression in higher organisms. *Science* 166:1474–1480.

WARNER, J. R., 1971. The assembly of ribosomes in yeast. *J. Biol. Chem.* 246:447–454.

WESSELLS, N. K., and F. H. WILT, 1965. Action of actinomycin D on exocrine pancreas cell differentiation. *J. Mol. Biol.* 13:767–779.

WILLIAMS, L. S., and F. C. NEIDHARDT, 1969. Synthesis and inactivation of aminoacyl-transfer RNA synthetases during growth of *Escherichia coli. J. Mol. Biol.* 43:529–550.

WIRTZ, K. W. D., and D. B. ZILVERSMIT, 1968. Exchange of phospholipids between liver mitrochondria and microsomes in vitro. *J. Biol. Chem.* 243:3596–3602.

WURTMAN, R. J., and J. AXELROD, 1967. Daily rhythmic changes in tyrosine transaminase activity of the rat liver. *Proc. Natl. Acad. Sci. USA* 57:1594–1598.

YAFFE, D., and M. FELDMAN, 1964. The effect of actinomycin D on heart and thigh muscle cells grown in vitro. *Devel. Biol.* 9:347–366.

YOSHIDA, A., G. STAMATOYANNOPOULOS, and A. MOTULSKY, 1967. Negro variant of glucose-6-phosphate dehydrogenase deficiency (A⁻) in man. *Science* 155:97–99.

72 Regulation and Importance of Intracellular Protein Degradation

ALFRED L. GOLDBERG

ABSTRACT In animal and bacterial cells, the rates of protein degradation can vary under different physiological conditions. For example, in skeletal muscle, contractile activity, hormones, and the supply of nutrients all affect protein degradation. Bacteria have proved highly useful for studying the mechanisms and significance of this process. During starvation, protein degradation in such cells increases several fold. Control of this response, which allows the cell to adapt to starvation, is coupled to the control of RNA synthesis. Cellular proteins vary widely in their rates of degradation, and cells selectively degrade abnormal or denatured proteins. These variations in the rates of degradation of specific proteins appear to reflect inherent differences in their sensitivity to endoproteases.

THE PROTEIN constituents of all cells, including those in the nervous system, are in a highly dynamic state. Whether found within organelles, in membranes, as structural components, or as soluble enzymes, cellular proteins are subject to continuous degradation and replacement through further synthesis (Schimke, 1970). The past 20 years have witnessed unprecedented advances in our knowledge about the synthesis of proteins. However, protein degradation is also of prime importance in determining intracellular amounts of enzymes or structural components. As yet we have only a rudimentary knowledge about the biochemical mechanisms, regulation and physiological significance of the degradative process.

A number of fundamental questions remain unanswered: (1) Why do different proteins in the same cell have distinct rates of turnover? (2) What physiological factors control overall rates of protein breakdown? (3) What enzymes are responsible for the turnover of cell proteins? (4) What might be the selective advantage to the organism of this continuous degradation of protein, which appears to be highly wasteful? Answers to these questions are not only of fundamental import to biochemists but also are highly relevant to a number of unsolved physiological problems. For example, in nerve cells the degradation of proteins must be intimately related to their axoplasmic flow, to the assembly and disassembly of membranes, and even to the mechanisms responsible for neuronal plasticity. The present chapter will attempt to review recent studies in my laboratory on the regulation and physiological significance of protein catabolism in animal and bacterial cells.

Protein turnover in growth and atrophy of muscle

Our own interest in protein breakdown arose out of studies into the biochemical mechanisms through which increased muscular activity causes hypertrophy and through which disuse causes atrophy (Goldberg, 1972c). Originally this research was undertaken as a model system for exploring how physiological function might regulate protein synthesis in an excitable tissue. These investigations unexpectedly raised the possibility that changes in the rates of protein catabolism might also contribute to cell growth and atrophy. Measurements of the fate of labeled proteins in rat muscle indicated that during atrophy the degradation of muscle proteins was augmented, while during compensatory growth the rates of degradation appeared to decrease (Goldberg, 1969). In both instances, the alterations in degradative rates appeared to have effects complementary to the changes occurring in the rates of protein synthesis (Table I).

These initial observations emphasized the necessity of learning more about the control of protein degradation for understanding the control of tissue size. Our initial studies, like most research in this area, estimated the proteolytic process from measurements of the loss of radioactive proteins from cells. Though valuable, this approach is awkward, expensive, and rather inappropriate for studies of mechanism of turnover; in addition it is subject to serious complications (e.g., the reincorporation of radioactive amino acids back into cell proteins). Recently Mr. Richard Fulks and Dr. Jeanne Li in this laboratory (Fulks et al., 1973; Li and Goldberg, 1973) have developed a simple procedure for studying protein breakdown in rat muscles in vitro, which should also be applicable to other isolated tissues or to cultured cells.

Using this technique, we have found that a variety of other physiological variables that influence muscle size

ALFRED L. GOLDBERG Department of Physiology, Harvard Medical School, Boston, Massachusetts

TABLE I
Factors influencing protein turnover in skeletal muscle

	Synthesis	Degradation
Denervation atrophy	↓	↑
Compensatory hypertrophy	↑	↓
Growth hormone	↑	—
Cortisone (glucocorticoids)	↓	↑
Starvation	↓	↑
Insulin*	↑	↓
Glucose*	—	↓
Free fatty acids*	—	—
Amino acids*	↑	↓
Contraction*		↓
Passive stretch*		↓

*Direct effect demonstrated in vitro.

This summary includes previous in vivo measurements of protein turnover in muscle during atrophy and hypertrophy (Edlin et al., 1968) as well as more recent measurements on protein turnover in isolated skeletal muscle in vitro (Fulks et al., 1973; Li and Goldberg, 1973).

also influence rates of protein catabolism (Table I). For example, insulin, which has long been known to promote protein synthesis and growth of muscle, also inhibits protein breakdown in this tissue (Fulks et al., 1973). This hormone appears to have a similar effect in heart (Morgan et al., 1971a, b), liver (Mortimore and Mondon, 1970) and cultured hepatoma cells (Hershko and Tomkins, 1971). On the other hand, food deprivation, which leads to the mobilization of protein reserves in muscle, not only inhibits protein synthesis in this tissue but also promotes protein degradation (Li and Goldberg, 1973). Supply of nutrients such as glucose or amino acids to isolated muscle (Li and Goldberg, 1973) and liver (Mortimore and Mondon, 1970) can inhibit the degradative process. One recent finding of special interest to neurobiology is that repeated electrical stimulation of muscle somehow inhibits protein degradation (Li and Goldberg, 1973). Even passive stretch of muscle reduces catabolism of muscle proteins, and this effect appears of potential therapeutic import (Li and Goldberg, 1973). As yet, we are still only at the stage of defining the factors influencing overall rates of proteolysis, and we have little idea of how degradation of specific proteins is affected under these various conditions.

Although the mechanisms responsible for these effects on protein breakdown are completely unclear at present, it is interesting that the effects of nutrient supply, hormones, and muscular activity on degradation are immediate and can be demonstrated in the absence of protein synthesis (Fulks et al., 1973; Li and Goldberg, 1973). Thus within the organism, average rates of protein breakdown in specific cells, like the mean rates of protein synthesis, change from moment to moment in response to a variety of physiological signals.

Studies of protein degradation in microorganisms

Several years ago, in order to study the mechanisms of protein degradation more effectively, we began to investigate the control of protein catabolism in *Escherichia coli*. Bacteria offer the biochemist or physiologist enormous technical advantages. Furthermore, such organisms exquisitely control their rates of protein degradation. In fact, for many years, textbooks of bacteriology claimed that bacteria do not turn over their protein constituents, because early experiments were carried out in growing cells under conditions where the degradative process is maximally inhibited. About 20 years ago, Mandelstam (1960) demonstrated that when bacteria were deprived of a required nutrient (e.g. a carbon or nitrogen source or a required amino acid), the rate of degradation of cell proteins increased several fold. This increase in proteolysis represents a physiological adaptation to the poor environment and can be rapidly reversed by readministration of the required material (Figure 1). Protein degradation also increases when rapidly growing cells enter stationary phase. At such times, growth ceases, protein synthesis is reduced, and protein breakdown increased markedly. Dilution of such cultures into fresh medium causes the reinitiation of normal growth and a rapid inhibition of protein breakdown.

The nongrowing bacteria thus resemble nongrowing mammalian tissues, where protein synthesis and protein catabolism are equally matched. In addition, the responses of the bacteria to *step-up* and *step-down* conditions appear similar to those observed in growing and atrophying muscle. During rapid growth of both cells, protein degradation is minimized while protein and RNA synthesis are maximal. In the nongrowing cells, protein degradation is augmented while synthetic processes are reduced. In the atrophying tissues, degradative events increase even further and exceed protein synthesis. The generality of growth-dependent changes in degradation remains to be established, although analogous findings have now been made in perfused liver (Mortimore and Mondon, 1970), perfused heart (Morgan et al., 1971a, 1971b), regenerating kidney in vivo (unpublished), and cultured hepatoma cells (Hershko and Tomkins, 1971).

Our major interest in studying the bacterial system has been to clarify the cellular mechanisms underlying the changes in protein catabolism. Step-down conditions not only promote degradation but also lead to an increased ability of the cells to synthesize certain catabolic enzymes (Magasanik, 1970). An initially attractive hypothesis was that the accumulation of cyclic AMP in such cells (which

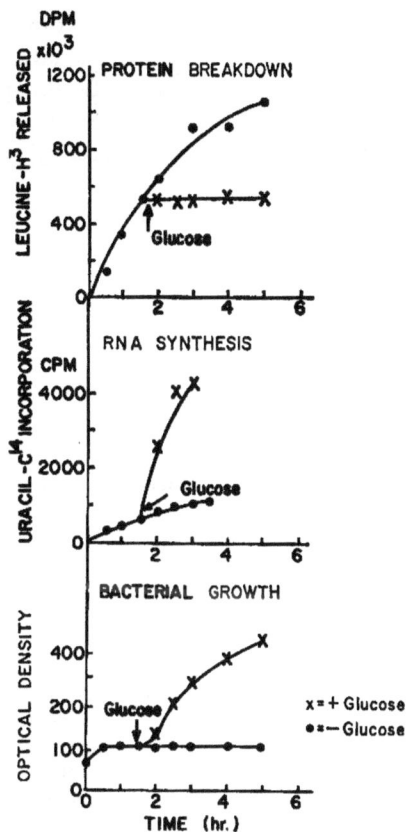

FIGURE 1 Effects of glucose deprivation on protein degradation, growth and RNA synthesis. *E. coli A33* was grown exponentially in glucose-minimal medium and ^{3}H-leucine for two generations. At time zero, they were deprived of the carbon source and the radioactive amino acid. The degradation of pre-existent proteins was measured from the release of ^{3}H-leucine (Goldberg, 1971) medium containing large amounts of non-radioactive leucine to prevent reutilization of the radioactive residues (Mandelstam, 1960). The RNA synthesis was measured by the incorporation of uracil-^{14}C into RNA by standard Millipore filter methods, and growth was followed with a Klett-Summerson Colorimeter. At 90 min, glucose was added back to the starved cultures.

promotes the synthesis of various catabolic enzymes) might also stimulate protein degradation (Perlman and Pastan, 1971). However, unpublished (Goldberg and Li, 1973) experiments with mutants in the cyclic AMP systems have discounted this view. In addition, the conditions affecting overall rates of protein catabolism also alter the synthesis of ribosomal and transfer RNA. Step-down markedly reduces RNA synthesis, while the supply of amino acids or glucose promotes RNA synthesis and inhibits protein catabolism (Figure 1). Various experiments in this laboratory have provided evidence that the control of protein degradation is in some way linked to the control of RNA synthesis.

Work in several laboratories has previously indicated that the production of ribosomal RNA is somehow dependent on the intracellular supply of aminoacyl tRNA (Edlin and Broda, 1968). The possibility that the supply of charged tRNA might also influence protein catabolism appeared attractive since it suggested a link between synthetic and degradative processes (Figure 2). Experiments were performed to determine whether the increased proteolysis during starvation resulted from a fall in the levels of amino acids or of charged tRNA (Goldberg and Li, 1973). One approach utilized bacterial strains which carried a specific temperature-sensitive aminoacyl tRNA synthetase. Such cells grow normally at the permissive temperature, but lack a specific species of aminoacyl tRNA at the nonpermissive temperature, growth ceases and rates of protein breakdown increases 8- to 12- fold (Goldberg and Li, 1973). Additional experiments using amino acid analogs to block selectively the synthesis of valyl-tRNA or agents that prevent formation of N-formyl methionyl-tRNA, also indicated that deprivation of a single charged tRNA can stimulate proteolysis (Goldberg and Li, 1973).

Unfortunately, we do not as yet understand the cellular mechanisms through which changes in the supply of charged tRNA might influence intracellular protein breakdown. Since the increased protein degradation occurred despite a profound inhibition of protein synthesis, it appears likely that this effect does not require the synthesis of new proteolytic enzymes. Instead, supply of nutrients through some effect on the levels of charged t RNA must influence the activity of proteases that exist in the growing cells. Control of protease activity can also explain the observation that readministration of nutrients to starved cells immediately reduced protein breakdown (Figure 1).

These experiments further support the conclusion that rates of protein breakdown are controlled coordinately with rates of RNA synthesis. All experimental conditions that were found to stimulate protein degradation (Goldberg and Li, 1973) have been reported previously to inhibit net RNA synthesis. Unfortunately, despite extensive investigation, we lack an adequate explanation for the control of ribosomal RNA synthesis. Mutants (*rel*) are known that fail to inhibit this process when the cells are starved for amino acids. Experiments by Sussman and Gilvarg (1969) and by us (unpublished) indicate that strains defective in regulating ribosome synthesis are also defective in stimulating protein breakdown on amino acid starvation. The *rel* mutation has also been found to influence glucose transport, nucleotide synthesis, and lipid metabolism. It appears likely that both protein breakdown and RNA synthesis depend on changes in some intermediary metabolite which affect a broad range

ALFRED L. GOLDBERG   829

of growth-related biochemical events. Such a pleiotropic control mechanism may also affect protein breakdown in mammalian cells (Goldberg and Li, 1973).

Inhibition of protein degradation

In order to learn more about biochemical pathways and the physiological significance of protein degradation, we attempted to find selective inhibitors of this process. A systematic attempt was made to test whether well-characterized inhibitors of proteolytic enzymes might also inhibit protein catabolism in starving bacteria. The most widespread type of proteolytic enzyme in nature is the serine protease, so designated because of a serine residue in its active sites which is particularly sensitive to attack by reagents such as diiosopropyl fluorophosphate (DFP) or the sulfonyl fluorides. These compounds selectively inactivate various well-known proteases, such as chymotrypsin or subtilisin, by covalently binding to this active-site serine. We found that such drugs also block the increased protein degradation occurring in starving *E. coli*. Most of our studies utilized the sulfonyl fluorides (PMSF and TSF) which unlike DFP are selective for proteases and are therefore relatively nontoxic. These agents can inhibit degradation in starving bacteria at concentrations that do not block cell growth (Prouty and Goldberg, 1972). In addition to the sulfonyl fluorides, several other inhibitors of pancreatic trypsin, such as the aromatic diamidines, also inhibit protein degradation in starving bacteria (Prouty and Goldberg, 1972).

These results suggest that a trypsin-like serine protease is responsible for the increased protein degradation in starving cells. Recent work in my laboratory has demonstrated the existence of such an enzyme in *E. coli*; however, it remains to be demonstrated whether this new protease is actually involved in protein degradation in vivo. Interestingly, these agents which are active in starved cells do not inhibit the low amount of protein degradation occurring in growing cells. These findings thus raise the possibility that *E. coli* contain two distinct proteolytic systems, possibly with different physiological functions: one active in growing cells and one activated during starvation.

Additional studies have supported the existence of two such systems, and these inhibitors have proved quite useful in studying their physiological importance. Mandelstam (1960) originally suggested that protein catabolism increases in poor environments in order that the cells can synthesize new enzymes appropriate to the new conditions. Unlike growing cells, which can synthesize required amino acids, cells deprived of a carbon or nitrogen source or a required amino acid can only obtain amino acids for synthesizing proteins from pre-existing cellular

proteins (Figure 2). This idea predicts that inhibitors of protein degradation during starvation should also block induction of new enzymes (Prouty and Goldberg, 1972). Starving cells can induce the enzyme β-galactosidase when administered the gratuitous inducer IPTG. How-

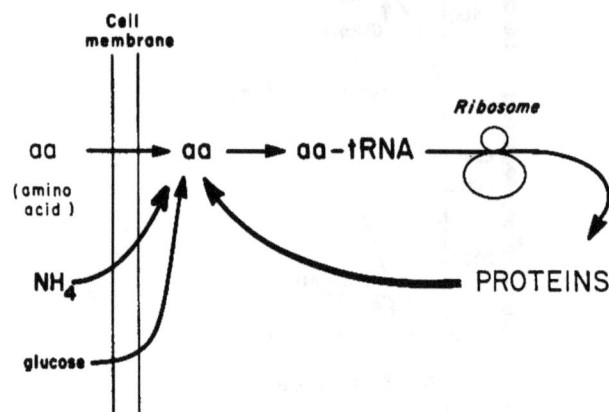

FIGURE 2 Relationship of protein degradation and protein synthesis. Growing cells obtain their amino acids from the surrounding medium or synthesize them from external sources of nitrogen and carbon. In poor environments, the starved cells obtain amino acids primarily from the increased protein degradation.

ever, when such cells are exposed to the sulfonyl fluorides or aromatic diamidines, induction of β-galactosidase was prevented (Figure 3). Administration of the required nutrients in the presence of the inhibitors once again permitted the synthesis of new enzymes. These results clearly demonstrate an adaptive role for protein breakdown in cells in poor environments. This situation appears highly reminiscent of the increased protein degradation that occurs in us mammals, where mobilization of body proteins is an important aspect of adaptation to starvation.

The degradation of abnormal proteins

These findings demonstrate an important adaptive role for the increased protein degradation in starving organisms, but they do not suggest a physiological function for the lower amount of protein breakdown seen in normal cells. It has often been naively suggested that intracellular protein degradation might serve to eliminate "proteinaceous waste" from the cell. According to this idea, proteins (like automobiles or humans) may also suffer from "wear and tear" processes and sooner or later denature. In order that such abnormal proteins do not accumulate, cells may have evolved enzymatic systems for their selective degradation. Although this idea appears

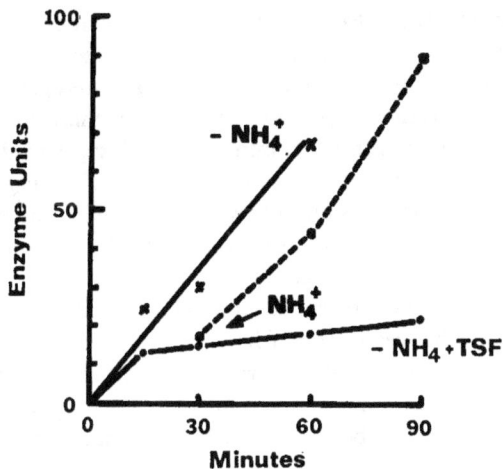

FIGURE 3 Importance of protein breakdown for induction of enzymes in cells deprived of nitrogen. *E. coli 19* was grown on glycerol-minimal medium and then deprived of a nitrogen source (NH_4^+). The nongrowing cells were administered isopropyl-β-D-thiogalactoside, a gratuitous inducer of β-galactosidase. This enzyme was synthesized presumably from amino acids supplied by protein breakdown. Toluene sulfonyl-fluoride (TSF), an inhibitor of protein breakdown during starvation (Prouty and Goldberg, 1972), greatly reduced enzyme induction, presumably by blocking the supply of amino acids. Readministration of ammonium chloride in the presence of TSF again permitted enzyme induction.

vague or even meaningless in chemical terms, it is in many ways an attractive hypothesis, and experiments were undertaken by Pine (1967) and ourselves (Goldberg, 1972a) to test whether cells can selectively degrade denatured proteins.

Proteins with abnormal conformations were produced by a variety of experimental approaches. For example, we studied the fate in growing bacteria of proteins that have incorporated amino acid analogs in place of the normal residues. As shown in Figure 4, proteins containing fluorophenylalanine or canavanine are catabolized more rapidly than normal cell constituents containing phenylalanine or arginine (Pine, 1967; Goldberg, 1972a). Altogether we have studied the effects of incorporation of 14 different analogs; all of them promote catabolism, although the effects of the various analogs on the rates of catabolism are quite different. Presumably those analogs that most disrupt normal conformations are most effective in promoting protein degradation.

In analogous experiments, we caused bacteria to produce unfinished polypeptide chains by administration of puromycin, which is incorporated into the growing polypeptide and causes its premature release from the ribosome. Proteins that have incorporated puromycin were found to be degraded much more quickly than the normal cell proteins (Pine, 1967; Goldberg, 1972a). Inde-

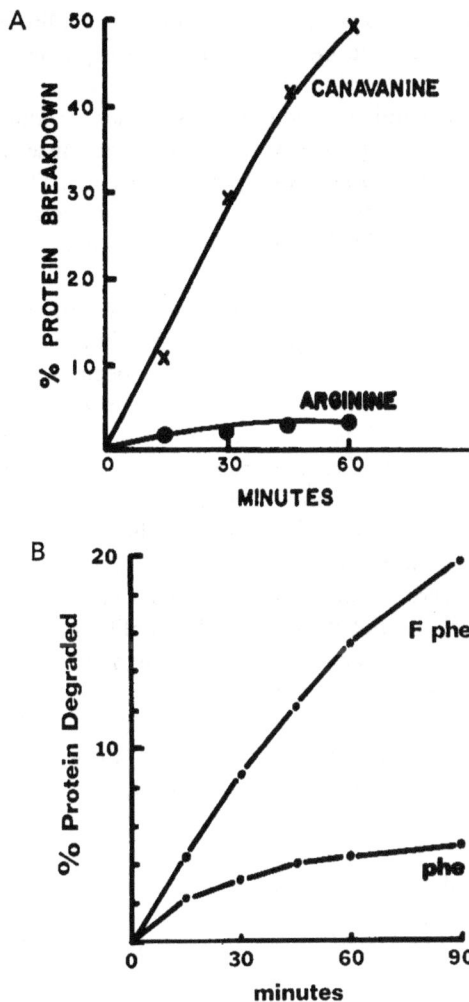

FIGURE 4 Degradation of proteins containing amino acid analogs in growing *E. coli*. (A) Compares the fate of proteins that have incorporated arginine or its analog canavanine; (B) Proteins that have incorporated phenylalanine or its analog fluorophenylalanine. Strain *A33*, an arginine-auxotroph (Figure 4A), or 83-5A, a phenylalanine-auxotroph (Figure 4B), were grown initially in glucose-minimal medium containing the required amino acids. They were then exposed to ^{3}H-leucine for five minutes in the presence of the natural amino acid or the analog. Cells were then transferred to nonradioactive medium containing normal amino acids. The rates of degradation of labeled proteins are expressed as the amount of ^{3}H-leucine released into acid-soluble form relative to that originally in proteins.

pendently of this work, two groups have obtained evidence that certain mutant proteins are rapidly catabolized, even though the wild-type proteins are perfectly stable (Platt et al., 1970; Goldschmidt, 1970). It appears likely that many other examples of this sort will be discovered in animal as well as bacterial cells.

Cells thus have the capacity to degrade aberrant proteins as might arise spontaneously through denaturation of cell enzymes or through genetic mutations. In addition, such proteins may also be formed as a consequence of mistakes in gene transcription or translation. To test this possibility, we studied bacterial strains that produce frequent mistakes in gene expression (e.g. the missense suppressors or the ribosomal ambiguity mutations). These experiments (Goldberg, 1972a) indicated that errors in protein synthesis lead to increased rates of protein catabolism.

The existence of a cellular mechanism for eliminating abnormal proteins would appear to be highly advantageous to the organism. It has frequently been argued (Goldberg and Wittes, 1966) that genetic mechanisms have evolved to minimize the harmful consequences of imprecise protein synthesis. Presumably, an enzymatic mechanism for eliminating abnormal or denatured proteins would be selected by evolution for similar reasons. The accumulation of "proteinaceous garbage" would be an especially serious threat to long-lived cells, such as neurons, which do not divide and thus unlike bacteria cannot dilute out denatured proteins through growth. It is interesting that several groups have presented evidence that cellular aging may result from increased production of abnormal proteins as a consequence of a faulty system for gene expression (Holliday and Tarrant, 1972). The continuous turnover of body constituents, though seemingly wasteful, by selectively removing proteins with abnormal conformations would serve to minimize such deleterious processes.

An implicit conclusion of this work is that the stability of a protein in vivo is influenced by its conformation which in turn must reflect its primary structure. Usually biochemists and geneticists have clearly distinguished between structural mutations, which influence enzymatic activity, and control-gene mutations that affect the concentrations of enzyme molecules. The finding that enzyme conformation may also be a major determinant of protein half lives thus gives an added significance to studies of tertiary structure.

Protein half lives and protease sensitivity

The finding that deviations from normal structure markedly influence protein stability in vivo implies that normal proteins share certain conformational features distinguishing them from abnormal proteins. How the cell might recognize and selectively degrade these abnormal proteins remains to be determined. The simplest model that one might draw to explain these findings would be that normal cells contain free proteases within the cytoplasm. Normal cell enzymes presumably share certain conformational features that have evolved to insure

relative resistance to these proteases. Deviations from these normal conformations might increase protease sensitivity. It is well documented that denatured proteins are more sensitive to proteolytic digestion than normal ones. The incorporation of amino acid analogs, the failure to complete polypeptides, or even the mistakes in gene transcription or translation might all augment the rate at which the resulting proteins are digested by proteolytic enzymes (Goldberg, 1972b).

In fact, we have obtained appreciable evidence for a correlation between protein half lives in vivo and their sensitivity in vitro to known proteases (Platt et al., 1970). The various treatments found to increase the intracellular rates of protein catabolism have all been found to increase sensitivity of the labeled proteins to well-characterized proteases such as trypsin or papain. These differences in protease sensitivity constitute further evidence for a conformational basis for differences in protein degradative rates.

These findings not only may explain the selective degradation of abnormal cell constituents but also raise the possibility that differences in protease sensitivity might contribute to the variation in half lives of normal proteins. It is now well documented that proteins within bacterial or mammalian cells vary markedly in their degradative rates; for example, in normal rat liver, half lives of specific enzymes are known to range from 11 min to 6 days (Schimke, 1970). We therefore tested whether a correlation might also exist between the in vivo stability of normal proteins and their sensitivity to known endoproteases (Goldberg, 1972b). To test this possibility, cells were administered a radioactive amino acid and either frozen immediately or allowed to grow for several generations and to turn over the labeled protein. In the frozen cells, a variety of cell proteins should be labeled; in the cells allowed to grow, those proteins with shorter half lives should be selectively lost and the proportion of label in protein constituents with long half lives should increase. Figure 5 demonstrates that the most stable proteins in vivo are on the average more resistant to trypsin than those that turn over more rapidly. Analogous findings were also obtained with other endopeptidases such as chymotrypsin, pronase or sublilisin.

Similar evidence has been obtained by us (Goldberg, 1973) and by Dice, Dehlinger, and Schimke (1973) for kidney, muscle, and tissue culture cells. In all these systems it was found that the more labile cell proteins are inherently more easily digested by proteases than more stable intracellular constituents. The structural features that distinguish the short-lived enzymes from more stable ones are unknown; presumably they are similar to but more subtle than the structural differences between nor-

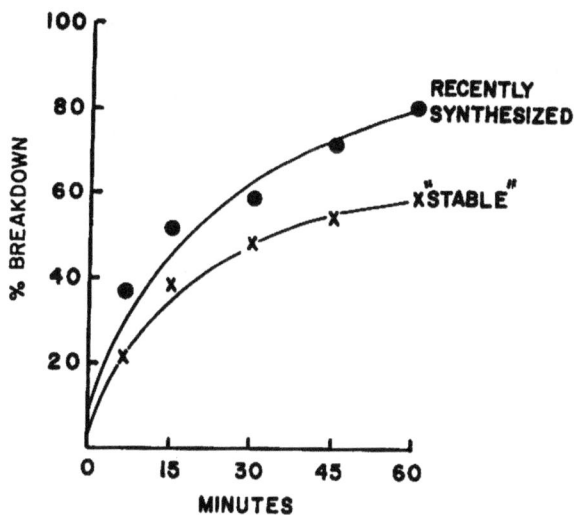

FIGURE 5 Comparison of trypsin sensitivity of *E. coli* proteins with different intracellular stabilities (Goldberg, 1972b). *E. coli A33* were exposed to ^{3}H-leucine for five minutes. Half the culture was frozen (recently synthesized) and the other half ("stable") grew for two generations in the presence of nonradioactive leucine, during which time the cells degraded 8% of the labeled proteins to acid-soluble form. These cells, which had lost the more labile cell proteins, were then frozen. The frozen cells were then lysed and treated with trypsin (100 μg/ml).

mal and abnormal proteins. In any case, the identification of conformational factors that determine protease sensitivity appears very important for understanding the regulation of enzyme levels.

Despite these extensive correlations, it appears quite unlikely that inherent differences in protease sensitivity by itself explains all the specificity in protein degradation. For example, we have been unable to demonstrate an increase in protease sensitivity of cellular proteins during starvation, even though overall protein breakdown increases at such times (Figure 1). The studies discussed above clearly suggest the activation of new proteolytic enzymes in starving cells (Figure 3). We believe these findings indicate that, although differences in protease sensitivity probably account for variations in half lives normally, physiological factors alter overall protein degradation by influencing the activity of proteolytic systems of the cell.

ACKNOWLEDGMENTS These studies were accomplished through the skill and cooperation of my colleagues: Mrs. Susan Martel, Mrs. Elizabeth Howell, Miss Patricia Ritchie, Dr. Jeanne Li, Mr. Richard Fulks, and Dr. Walter Prouty. I am grateful to the Air Force Office of Scientific Research and the Muscular Dystrophy Associations of America for their support of this research. Dr. Goldberg holds a Research Career Development Award from the National Institute of Neurological Diseases and Stroke.

REFERENCES

DICE, F., P. J. DEHLINGER, and R. T. SCHIMKE, 1973. Studies on the correlation between size and relative degradation rate of soluble proteins. *J. Biol. Chem.* (in press).

EDLIN, G., and P. BRODA, 1968. Physiology and genetics of the "ribonucleic acid control" locus in *Escherichia coli. Bact. Rev.* 32:206–226.

FULKS, R., J. B. LI, and A. L. GOLDBERG, 1973. Effects of insulin and glucose on protein breakdown in isolated rat diaphragm. *J. Biol. Chem.* (in press).

GOLDBERG, A. L., and R. E. WITTES, 1966. Genetic code: Aspects of organization. *Science* 153:420–424.

GOLDBERG, A. L., 1969. Protein turnover in skeletal muscle. I, II. *J. Biol. Chem.* 244:3217–3222; 3223–3229.

GOLDBERG, A. L., 1971. A role for aminoacyl-tRNA in the regulation of protein catabolism in *Escherichia coli. Proc. Natl. Acad. Sci. USA* 68:362–366.

GOLDBERG, A. L., 1972a. Degradation of "abnormal" proteins in *E. coli. Proc. Nat. Acad. Sci. USA* 69:422–426.

GOLDBERG, A. L., 1972b. Correlation between rates of degradation of bacterial proteins in vivo and their sensitivity to proteases. *Proc. Nat. Acad. Sci. USA* 69:2640–2644.

GOLDBERG, A. L., 1972c. Mechanisms of growth and atrophy of skeletal muscle. In *Muscle Biology.* New York: Marcel Dekker, pp. 81–118.

GOLDBERG, A. L., 1973. Further evidence for a correlation between protease-sensitivity and protein degradative rates in animal and bacterial cells. *J. Biol. Chem.* (in press).

GOLDBERG, A. L., and J. B. LI, 1973. Physiological significance of protein breakdown in animal and bacterial cells. *Fed. Proc.* (in press).

GOLDSCHMIDT, R., 1970. In vivo degradation of nonsense fragments in *E. coli. Nature (London)* 228:1151–1156.

HERSHKO, A., and G. M. TOMKINS, 1971. Studies on the degradation of tyrosine aminotransferase in hepatoma cells in culture. *J. Biol. Chem.* 246:710–714.

HOLLIDAY, R., and G. TARRANT, 1972. Altered enzymes in aging human fibroblasts. *Nature (London)* 238:26–30.

LI, J. B., and A. L. GOLDBERG, 1973. Factors affecting protein degradation in skeletal muscle. *J. Biol. Chem.* (in press).

MAGASANIK, B., 1970. Glucose effects: Inducer exclusion and repression. In *The Lactose Operon*, J. B. Beckwith and D. Zipser, eds. New York: Cold Spring Harbor Laboratory, pp. 189–219.

MANDELSTAM, J., 1960. The intracellular turnover of protein and nucleic acids and its role in biochemical differentiation. *Bact. Rev.* 24:289–308.

MORGAN, H. E., D. C. N. EARL, A. BROADUS, E. B. WOLPERT, K. E. GIGER, and L. S. JEFFERSON, 1971a. Regulation of protein synthesis in heart muscle. I. Effect of amino acid levels on protein synthesis. *J. Biol. Chem.* 246:2152–2162.

MORGAN, H. E., L. S. JEFFERSON, E. B. WOLPERT, and D. E. RANNELS, 1971b. Regulation of protein synthesis in heart muscle. II. Effect of amino acid levels and insulin on ribosomal aggregation. *J. Biol. Chem.* 246:2163–2170.

MORTIMORE, G. E., and C. E. MONDON, 1970. Inhibition by insulin of valine turnover in liver. *J. Biol. Chem.* 245:2375–2383.

PERLMAN, R. L., and I. PASTAN, 1971. The role of cyclic AMP in bacteria. In *Current Topics in Cellular Regulation.* New York: Academic Press, pp. 117–134.

PINE, M. J., 1967. Response of intracellular proteolysis to

alteration of bacterial protein and the implications in metabolic regulation. *J. Bact.* 93:1527–1533.

PLATT, T., J. MILLER, and J. WEBER, 1970. In vivo degradation of mutant Lac repressor. *Nature (London)* 228:1154–1156.

PROUTY, W. F., and A. L. GOLDBERG, 1972. Inhibitors of protein degradation in *E. coli* and their physiological effects. *J. Biol. Chem.* 247:3341–3352.

SCHIMKE, R. T., 1970. Regulation of protein degradation in mammalian tissues. *Mammalian Protein Metabolism.* 4:177–228. (See also R. T. Schimke, this volume.)

SUSSMAN, A. J., and C. GILVARG, 1969. Protein turnover in amino acid-starved strains of *Escherichia coli* K-12 differing in their ribonucleic acid control. *J. Biol. Chem.* 244:6304–6306.

73 Regulation of Riboflavin Metabolism by Thyroid Hormone

RICHARD S. RIVLIN

ABSTRACT Physiological amounts of thyroid hormone enhance the conversion of riboflavin to the two coenzymes, flavin mononucleotide (FMN) and flavin adenine dinucleotide (FAD). Biochemical similarities exist between hypothyroid and riboflavin-deficient animals with respect to activities of FMN-requiring and FAD-requiring enzymes and concentrations of tissue flavins. Diminished responsiveness to thyroid hormone is demonstrable in riboflavin deficiency. In liver and in brain of newborn animals, thyroid hormone accelerates the development of the FAD-synthesizing enzyme, FAD pyrophosphorylase. By increasing flavin synthesis, thyroid hormone has a potential role in increasing the availability of FAD for a number of flavoprotein enzymes during development. Thyroid hormone regulates riboflavin metabolism, and riboflavin, in turn, appears to regulate certain aspects of thyroid hormone action.

CHANGES IN THE activities of certain key enzymes in the nervous system may have important implications for the metabolism of the brain as a whole. A recurrent theme in this part is that enzyme activities may be altered by a change either in the rate of synthesis or in the rate of degradation, and furthermore that small molecules may alter the conformational structure of the enzyme and, thereby, exert profound influences upon catalytic activity. These principles are highly relevant to the study of a specific aspect of the regulation of brain function, namely, the thyroid hormonal control of riboflavin metabolism.

It will be recalled that the metabolic role of riboflavin resides largely in its being the precursor of flavin mononucleotide (FMN) and flavin adenine dinucleotide (FAD), two coenzymes that are required for a wide variety of important biochemical reactions (Rivlin, 1970a, 1970b). FMN and FAD not only are required for catalysis, but they also confer stability upon the flavoprotein apoenzymes to which they are bound. Compared to the flavoprotein holoenzymes, most apoenzymes exhibit some degree of lability with respect to heat denaturation, changes in ionic strength, exposure to various reagents such as cadmium chloride and mercuric acetate, or to other treatments (Neims and Weimar, 1973). Among the flavoprotein enzymes that have been studied most thoroughly in this fashion are included lipoamide dehydrogenase (Kalse and Veegar, 1968), D-amino acid oxidase (Dixon and Kleppe, 1965), glutathione reductase (Staal et al., 1969), and glucose oxidase (Swoboda, 1969).

Much attention has been directed toward investigating the stimulation of apoenzyme synthesis by thyroid hormone (Barker, 1951; Sokoloff et al., 1968; Tata, 1964; Wolff and Wolff, 1964) but relatively little attention toward studying the control of coenzyme synthesis. Evidence has accumulated indicating that thyroid hormone regulates the synthesis of the flavin coenzymes, enhancing the hepatic conversion of riboflavin to both FMN and FAD (Rivlin, 1970a). Hepatic concentrations of FMN and FAD in hypothyroid rats are reduced to one-third of those of normal animals and are restored to normal by treatment with thyroxine (Domjan and Kokai, 1966; Rivlin and Langdon, 1966). In this chapter, current knowledge concerning the hormonal control of flavin synthesis, especially in relation to brain function, is reviewed.

By regulating the rate of synthesis of the coenzyme moieties, thyroid hormone may determine the activities of many flavoprotein enzymes of biological importance. Studies have been recently performed in rat liver on three of the four enzymes involved in the riboflavin-to-FAD pathway. An important site of thyroid hormone control appears to be flavokinase, the enzyme catalyzing the initial conversion of riboflavin to FMN. Of the enzymes investigated, flavokinase undergoes the largest quantitative increase in activity after administration of thyroid hormone and, also, is the only enzyme of the group that decreases in activity in hypothyroidism. Of particular importance is that physiological doses of thyroid hormone are effective as enzyme inducers of flavokinase. Thyroid hormone also causes smaller increases in the activities of FAD pyrophosphorylase, which converts FMN to FAD, and of FMN phosphatase, which degrades FMN to riboflavin (Rivlin, 1970a, 1970b). The thyroid hormonal regulation of FMN and FAD synthesis and the role of these coenzymes in stabilizing the flavoprotein apoenzymes are shown diagrammatically in Figure 1.

RICHARD S. RIVLIN College of Physicians and Surgeons of Columbia University, New York

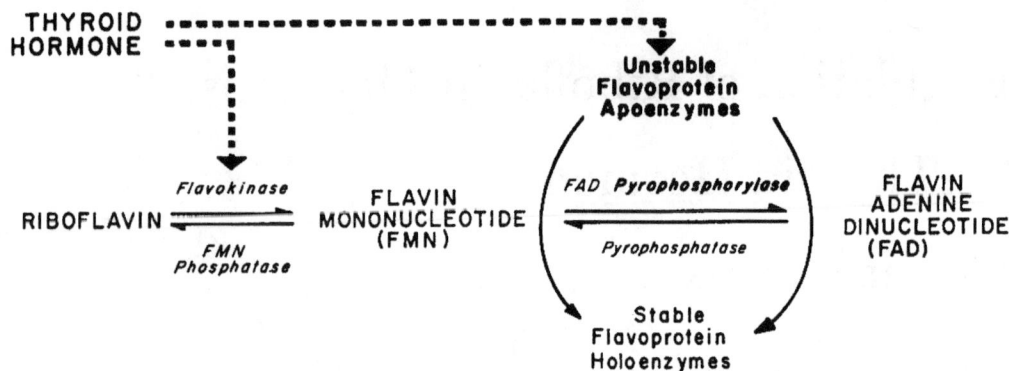

FIGURE 1 Diagrammatic representation of the postulated role of thyroid hormone in enhancing the biosynthesis of flavoprotein apoenzymes and of the coenzymes FMN and FAD (Rivlin, 1970a).

The nature of the increase in activity of flavokinase produced by thyroid hormone is complex and is not completely understood. Treatment with actinomycin D does not block the increase in enzyme activity (Rivlin, 1970b). Results of studies in vitro suggest that the thyroxine-induced increase in flavokinase activity may be due at least in part to a decrease in the rate of enzyme inactivation. When normal liver is homogenized, centrifuged at 100,000 × g for 1 hr, and then incubated in buffer at 37°C, flavokinase activity is rapidly lost. From 0 to 30 min after the start of incubation, there is very little change in enzyme activity; after 30 min, however, enzyme activity decreases in a sharp and nearly linear fashion. Ninety minutes after the start of incubation, there is loss of almost all enzyme activity (Rivlin, 1969b).

A striking difference is observed between enzyme from normal and hyperthyroid animals in the loss of activity that occurs during incubation under these conditions. As shown in Figure 2, enzyme from hyperthyroid animals is inactivated at a much slower rate than that obtained from normal animals: After 90 min of incubation, nearly 75% of the original activity has been preserved. Further experiments were conducted in which tissue extracts were passed through a Sephadex G 25 column, a procedure that results in the removal of molecules of less than 5000 mol wt. The tissue extracts following column chromatography were incubated in a similar fashion to that described above. A marked loss of stability of the enzyme from euthyroid and especially from hyperthyroid animals was noted. These preliminary observations suggest that the greater stability of the enzyme from hyperthyroid than from normal animals is due not to an inherent property of the enzyme protein but more likely to the presence of increased quantities of one or more small molecules that stabilize the enzyme (Rivlin, 1969b). The delayed inactivation of the enzyme from hyperthyroid animals in vitro raises the possibility that increased enzyme activity observed in animals treated with thyroid hormone may be due at least in part to a decrease in the rate of enzyme degradation.

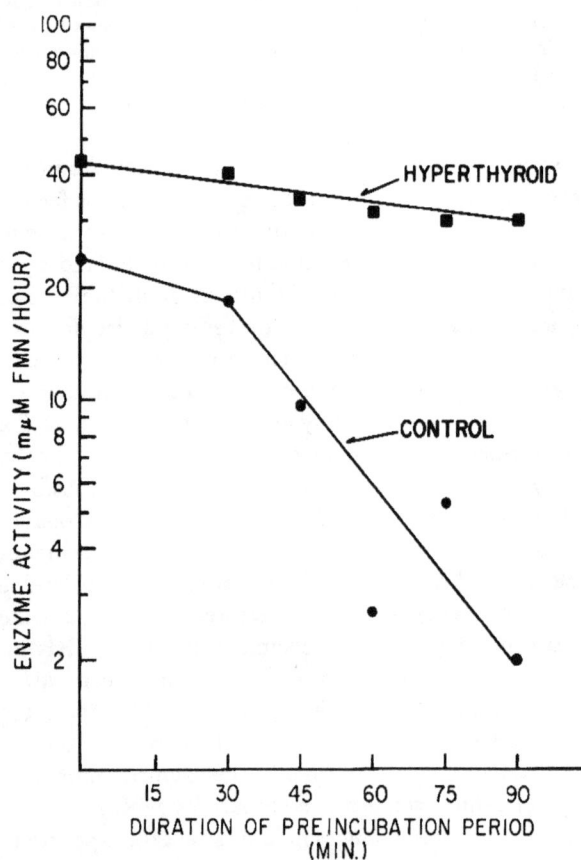

FIGURE 2 Differential rates of inactivation in vitro of hepatic flavokinase obtained from normal and hyperthyroid animals. Experiments were performed using supernatant solutions derived from centrifugation of liver homogenates at 100,000 × g for 1 hour. Enzymes were incubated at 37° C in buffer for periods from 0 to 90 min (reproduced from Rivlin, 1969b).

Certain biochemical measurements in hypothyroidism bear a remarkable similarity to those of riboflavin deficiency. These include at least three parameters: (1) hepatic concentrations of FAD, FMN, and free riboflavin, (2) activities of a number of FMN- and FAD-requiring enzymes, such as xanthine oxidase and D-amino acid oxidase, and (3) activities of the enzymes which are involved in the biosynthesis and degradation of FMN and FAD. Thus, hepatic flavin concentrations and activities of flavoprotein enzymes are largely decreased both in hypothyroidism and in riboflavin deficiency. Hepatic flavokinase activity is diminished and that of FMN phosphatase is unchanged in both conditions. The biochemical changes in hypothyroidism tend generally to be in the same direction as those of riboflavin deficiency but are of lesser magnitude (Rivlin, 1970b).

In addition to resembling hypothyroidism in certain respects, riboflavin deficiency results in diminished responsiveness to thyroid hormone. The induction of mitochondrial α-glycerophosphate dehydrogenase, an FAD-requiring enzyme, by triiodothyronine (T_3) is greatly diminished in riboflavin-deficient rats (Rivlin and Wolf, 1969). In normal animals, administration of triiodothyronine in a single large dose results in a 10-fold increase in enzyme activity measured 48 hr later. Triiodothyronine given similarly to hypothyroid animals increases enzyme activity 75-fold. By contrast, T_3 administration to riboflavin-deficient animals increases enzyme activity only 5-fold. Both the basal activity and the activity induced by T_3 closely parallel the decline in the tissue concentration of FAD with increasing duration of riboflavin deficiency, as shown in Figure 3. Normal enzyme induction can be restored to deficient rats by feeding riboflavin for several days, even when the intake of food is limited concurrently. Similar findings are not observed when caloric intake alone is decreased. In animals that have been starved for 3 to 5 days, both the basal and the T_3-induced activities of mitochondrial α-glycerophosphate dehydrogenase are entirely normal (Wolf and Rivlin, 1970). Riboflavin deficiency also decreases the hepatic deiodination of thyroxine (Galton and Ingbar, 1965). It is likely that the decreased hepatic activities of mitochondrial α-glycerophosphate dehydrogenase, both basal activity and that induced by thyroid hormone, may be related to the lack of FAD available for stabilizing newly synthesized apoenzyme proteins.

Studies of the regulation of riboflavin metabolism have been extended to the perinatal period. These investigations derived their impetus from the previous knowledge that as a group the FMN- and FAD-requiring enzymes, such as TPN-cytochrome C reductase and xanthine oxidase, as well as the tissue levels of FMN and FAD, have a characteristic pattern of development. At the time of

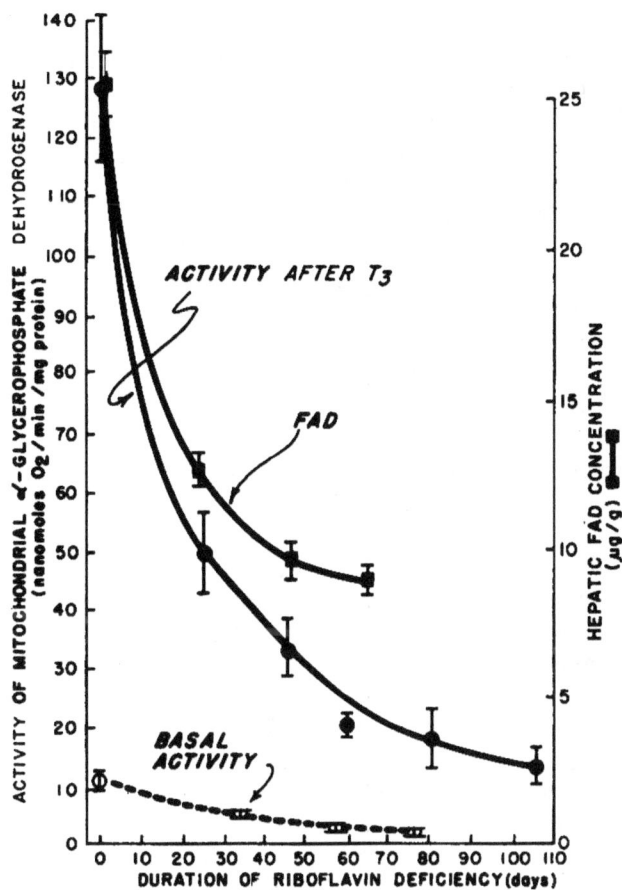

FIGURE 3 Basal and triiodothyronine-induced activities of mitochondrial α-glycerophosphate dehydrogenase and hepatic concentrations of FAD expressed as a function of duration of riboflavin deficiency. [Data are expressed as mean ± 1 SEM and have been obtained in part from Wolf and Rivlin (1970).]

birth, low but measureable concentrations of FMN and FAD and activities of FMN- and FAD-requiring enzymes are found and by the time of weaning at 21 days, adult or nearly adult levels have been attained (Burch et al., 1958). This sequence of events that occurs during postnatal development likely reflects the mutual interdependence of the flavoprotein enzymes and their coenzymes, FMN and FAD, because each is required for the stabilization of the other.

The enzymes involved in FMN and FAD biosynthesis, namely flavokinase and FAD pyrophosphorylase, undergo biochemical maturation much earlier than either the tissue coenzymes levels or the activities of flavoprotein enzymes. The major increases in hepatic flavokinase and FAD pyrophosphorylase activities occur shortly before birth. At the time of birth, levels similar to that of adults are already demonstrable (Rivlin, 1969a). The fact that the fetal thyroid gland in rats first begins to function late in gestation (Nataf et al., 1971) raises the possibility that thyroid hormone may be an important stimulus to the prenatal acceleration of development of these enzymes. Similarly, Greengard (1969) noted that thyroxine administration in gestation markedly accelerated the development of glucose-6-phosphatase and of arginase activities in fetal liver.

It was of interest to inquire whether thyroid hormone accelerates FAD synthesis during the perinatal period. Experiments were performed in which newborn animals received subcutaneous injections of L-thyroxine, 10 μg/animal, every other day for 8 days. In these animals hepatic FAD pyrophosphorylase activity was increased 35% above that of animals similarly treated with saline. Increases in FAD pyrophosphorylase activity were also observed in animals which had received thyroxine for only three days. The magnitude of these thyroxine-induced increases in hepatic enzyme activity in newborn animals is entirely comparable to that observed in adult animals (Rivlin and Hornibrook, 1971a).

Another system in which thyroid hormone is critical for normal development is the metamorphosing tadpole, *Rana catesbiana*. In the absence of thyroid hormone, tadpoles will not undergo metamorphosis, and will remain in an immature state. When tadpoles are treated with exogenous thyroid hormone, acceleration of metamorphosis occurs (Etkin, 1964). Immersion of tadpoles in a solution of thyroxine at 10^{-8} M for 6 to 11 days does not appear to influence hepatic FAD pyrophosphorylase activity, but if treatment is continued for 15 to 23 days, a significant increase (p < 0.01) in enzyme activity occurs. FAD pyrophosphorylase under these conditions is increased from 0.245 $\pm$ 0.018 mμM FAD/mg protein/hr to 0.357 $\pm$ 0.020. These findings indicate that changes in the activity of an FAD biosynthetic enzyme accompany thyroxine-induced metamorphosis (Fass et al., 1971).

The regulation of riboflavin metabolism in the developing tadpole is being studied further with structural analogues of riboflavin, each compound containing one or more substitutions on the isoalloxazine ring. The riboflavin analogues were generously provided by Merck & Co. Groups of tadpoles in premetamorphosis were injected three times a week with 13 μg of each of 14 analogues of riboflavin, and were observed for more than 4 months. The solubility of the analogues was a major factor in determining the dosage. Each tadpole was in an individual beaker containing 300 cc of standing tap water.

During the 4 month interval, tadpoles that had been injected with saline only underwent considerable morphological changes, with the development first of hind legs, followed by forelegs and atrophy of the tail. The hind limb length to tail length ratio, a simple, accurate, and widely accepted index of metamorphosis (Etkin, 1964),

increased in normal animals from approximately 0 to nearly 1.0. By contrast, in each group of analogue-treated tadpoles, a degree of interference with tadpole metamorphosis was demonstrable. Some compounds had a relatively small effect upon the hind limb length to tail length ratio, while others almost completely blocked metamorphosis. Four weeks after the start of treatment with analogues of riboflavin, these effects were already demonstrable and became more apparent with increasing duration of treatment (Rivlin et al., 1972).

A more rapid inhibition of metamorphosis can be demonstrated when tadpoles that had been placed in a solution of 2×10^{-8} M thyroxine for 2 to 3 weeks simultaneously received injections of analogues of riboflavin. Results of a typical experiment are shown in Table I.

TABLE I

Effects of treatment with an analogue* of riboflavin upon thyroxine-induced metamorphosis in tadpoles

Treatment Group	Number of Tadpoles	Hind Limb Length/Tail-Length Ratio	
		Before Treatment	14 Days After Treatment
1. Thyroxine	10	0.07 $\pm$ 0.02	0.56 $\pm$ 0.03
2. Analogue + Thyroxine	10	0.09 $\pm$ 0.02	0.33 $\pm$ 0.04

Data are expressed as mean $\pm$ 1 SEM.

*6-chloro-9-(1'-D-dulcityl) isoalloxazine. Each treated animal received an intraperitoneal injection of 13 μg dissolved in isotonic saline three times per week.

Animals were individually immersed in 300 cc solution of 2×10^{-8}M thyroxine dissolved in standing tap water.

Significance of difference between groups 1 and 2 before treatment = p > 0.05, and after treatment = p < 0.001.

(Data have been obtained from Rivlin et al., 1972.)

Tadpoles received thrice weekly injections of 6-chloro-9-(1'-D-dulcityl) isoalloxazine while immersed in thyroxine, and comparative measurements were made with a group of thyroxine-treated animals that had not received injections of this analog. In animals treated with thyroxine together with the riboflavin analog, the hind limb length to tail length ratio increased only half as much as in animals treated with thyroxine alone. Studies with other analogues of riboflavin have yielded similar results, with considerable variability in the degree of inhibition of metamorphosis (Rivlin et al., 1972).

These findings in mammals and in amphibia provide the background for current studies which are examining riboflavin metabolism in the developing rat brain. Thyroid hormone is known to regulate the early development of the brain, stimulating the synthesis of brain proteins and the deposition of myelin. During the critical period of its growth and development, the brain undergoes an increase in oxygen consumption and protein synthesis under thyroid hormone stimulation. After brain maturation has been achieved, thyroid hormone will no longer increase oxygen consumption or protein synthesis (Eayrs, 1971; Balazs et al., 1971; Sokoloff and Roberts, 1971).

Hormonal regulation of FAD synthesis during the critical period of brain development could play a potentially important role in stabilizing the newly synthesized apoenzyme moieties of a large number of flavoproteins. In the hypothyroid brain, the activities of certain FAD-dependent enzymes, notably succinic dehydrogenase, are reduced (Hamburgh and Flexner, 1957; Garcia Argiz et al., 1967). A possible lack of FAD available for conferring stability upon labile flavoprotein apoenzymes could be one of a number of mechanisms accounting for the deleterious effects of early hypothyroidism upon brain function.

To determine whether FAD synthesis in newborn brains is subject to hormonal control, animals within 24 hr of birth were injected with thyroxine, 10 μg/animal, each day or every other day for 8 days. To control nutritional factors and to minimize differences among animals, litter sizes were kept constant at 8 animals, half of which received thyroxine and half isotonic saline. Mothers were rotated daily among the litters in each experiment. Specimens of cerebrum promptly removed after sacrifice were assayed for FAD pyrophosphorylase activity. In newborn animals, enzyme activity in cerebrum was approximately half that in liver expressed per gram wet weight

and had a lower magnesium requirement than the enzyme in liver. FAD pyrophosphorylase activity in the cerebrum of saline-treated control rats was 15.1 ± 1.0 mμ mole FAD formed/g fresh weight/hour. Enzyme activity in thyroxine-treated animals of 21.3 ± 1.9 was significantly greater ($p < 0.01$) than in controls and was similar to the activity in the brain of adult animals.

Although FAD pyrophosphorylase could be increased in activity in liver of newborn animals by treatment with thyroxine for only 3 days, this time period was not sufficient to increase enzyme activity in the cerebrum of these animals (Rivlin and Hornibrook, 1971b). As shown in Table II, thyroxine administration was effective in increasing FAD pyrophosphorylase activity in the cerebrum of newborn animals but did not appear to increase enzyme activity in the cerebrum of adult animals. This finding is compatible with previous observations referred to above documenting the resistance of the adult brain to regulation by thyroid hormone (Sokoloff and Roberts, 1971). It appears that thyroid hormone may indeed regulate the availability of FAD for developing enzyme systems in the newborn brain.

Measurements of the conversion of ^{14}C-riboflavin to ^{14}C-FMN and ^{14}C-FAD in vivo provide additional evidence for the regulatory role of thyroid hormone. Radioactive flavins are being separated and quantitated using newly devised methods of isotope dilution and ion exchange column chromatography with DEAE-Sephadex A-25 (Fazekas, 1973). The results of recently obtained measurements in adult liver suggest that the magnitudes of the changes in flavokinase and in FAD pyrophosphorylase activity produced by both hyper- and hypothyroidism are similar to the magnitude of the changes in the rates of ^{14}C-FMN and ^{14}C-FAD synthesis from ^{14}C-riboflavin in vivo. Preliminary findings in the brains of newborn animals suggest that the magnitudes of increases in FAD pyrophosphorylase activity and in ^{14}C-FAD synthesis produced thyroxine are nearly identical. In brains of adult rats, neither enzyme activity nor ^{14}C-FAD synthesis is augmented by thyroxine. Studies are in progress to determine whether vitamin utilization is impaired in the brains of hypothyroid animals. In view of the increasing evidence (Eichenwald and Fry, 1969; Winick, 1970) that malnutrition during fetal and postnatal life has critical effects upon brain development, it may be important to consider that endogenous factors such as hormones may also regulate the nutritional status of the developing brain.

TABLE II

Effects of thyroxine treatment of newborn and adult male rats upon FAD pyrophosphorylase activity in cerebrum

Treatment Group	Age at Sacrifice (days)	Number of Animals	FAD Pyrophosphorylase Activity (mμ mole FAD formed/ g fresh wt/hr)
1. Saline	8	11 litters*	15.1 ± 1.0
2. Thyroxine	8	11 litters*	21.2 ± 1.5
3. Saline	67	28	22.5 ± 0.9
4. Thyroxine	67	21	25.2 ± 1.8

Data are expressed as mean ± 1 SEM.

*In each litter of newborn animals, half received thyroxine, 10 μg/animal, s.c. every day or every other day, and half received isotonic saline for 8 days; adults received thyroxine and saline on a similar weight basis.

Significance of difference between saline and thyroxine groups in 8 day old group = $p < 0.01$, and in 67 day old group = $p > 0.05$.

(Data are derived in part from Rivlin and Hornibrook, 1971b.)

ACKNOWLEDGMENTS This work was supported in part by USPHS Grants AM 15265 and CA 12126, and by grants from the Stella and Charles Guttman Foundation, Inc. and the National Association for Mental Health, Inc.

RICHARD S. RIVLIN   839

REFERENCES

Balazs, R., W. A. Cocks, J. T. Eayrs, and S. Kovacs, 1971. Biochemical effects of thyroid hormones on the developing brain. In *Hormones in Development*, M. Hamburgh and E. J. W. Barrington, eds. New York: Appleton-Century-Crofts, pp. 357–379.

Barker, S. B., 1951. Mechanism of action of the thyroid hormone. *Physiol. Rev.* 31:205–243.

Burch, H. B., O. H. Lowry, T. De Gubareff, and S. R. Lowry, 1958. Flavin enzymes in liver and kidney of rats from birth to weaning. *J. Cell Comp. Physiol.* 52:503–510.

Dixon, M., and K. Kleppe, 1965. D-amino acid oxidase. I. Dissociation and recombination of the holoenzyme. *Biochem. Biophys. Acta* 96:357–367.

Domjan, G., and K. Kokai, 1966. The flavin adenine dinucleotide (FAD) content of the rat's liver in hypothyroid state and in the liver of hypothyroid animals after in vivo thyroxine treatment. *Acta Biol. Acad. Sci. Hung.* 16:237–241.

Eayrs, J. T., 1971. Thyroid and developing brain: Anatomical and behavioral effects. In *Hormones in Development*, M. Hamburgh and E. J. W. Barrington, eds. New York: Appleton-Century-Crofts, pp. 345–355.

Eichenwald, H. F., and P. C. Fry, 1969. Nutrition and learning. *Science* 163:644–648.

Etkin, W., 1964. Metamorphosis. In *Physiology of the Amphibia*, J. A. Moore, ed. New York: Academic Press, pp. 427–468.

Fass, S., M. Osnos, R. Hornibrook, and R. S. Rivlin, 1971. Effects of thyroxine on hepatic FAD pyrophosphorylase activity in tadpoles. *Program of the Forty-Seventh Meeting of the American Thyroid Association*, p. 42 (abstract).

Fazekas, A. G., 1973. Chromatographic and radioisotopic methods for the analysis of riboflavin and the flavin coenzymes. In *Riboflavin*, R. S. Rivlin, ed. New York: Appleton Century Crofts (in press).

Galton, V. A., and S. H. Ingbar, 1965. Effects of vitamin deficiency on the in vitro and in vivo deiodination of thyroxine in the rat. *Endocrinology* 77:169–176.

Garcia Argiz, C. A., J. M. Pasquini, B. Kaplun, and C. J. Gomez, 1967. Hormonal regulation of brain development. II. Effect of neonatal thyroidectomy on succinate dehydrogenase and other enzymes in developing cerebral cortex and cerebellum of the rat. *Brain Res.* 6:635–646.

Greengard, O., 1969. Analogies between mammalian and amphibian biochemical differentiation; the role of thyroxine. In *Advances in Enzyme Regulation*, Vol. 7, G. Weber, ed. Oxford: Pergamon Press, pp. 283–289.

Hamburgh, M., and L. B. Flexner, 1957. Biochemical and physiological differentiation during morphogenesis. XXI. Effect of hypothyroidism and hormone therapy on enzyme activities of the developing cerebral cortex of the rat. *J. Neurochem.* 1:279–288.

Kalse, J. F., and C. Veeger, 1968. Relation between conformations and activities of lipoamide dehydrogenase. I. Relation between diaphorase and lipoamide dehydrogenase activities upon binding of FAD by the apoenzyme. *Biochim. Biophys. Acta* 159:244–256.

Nataf, B. M., J. Harel, and J. Imbenotte, 1971. Effect of thyrotropic hormone on thyroid glands of the fetal and newborn rat. In *Hormones in Development*, M. Hamburgh and E. J. W. Barrington, eds. New York: Appleton-Century-Crofts, pp. 781–792.

Neims, A. H., and W. R. Weimar, 1973. Physical and chemical properties of flavins; Binding of flavins to protein and conformational effects; Biosynthesis of riboflavin. In *Riboflavin*, R. S. Rivlin, ed. New York: Appleton-Century-Crofts (in press).

Rivlin, R. S., 1969a. Perinatal development of enzymes synthesizing FMN and FAD. *Amer. J. Physiol.* 216:979–982.

Rivlin, R. S., 1969b. Thyroid hormone and the adolescent growth spurt: clinical and fundamental consideration. In *Adolescent Nutrition and Growth*, F. Heald, ed. New York: Appleton-Century-Crofts, pp. 235–252.

Rivlin, R. S., 1970a. Medical progress: Riboflavin metabolism, *New Eng. J. Med.* 283:463–472.

Rivlin, R. S., 1970b. Regulation of flavoprotein enzymes in hypothyroidism and in riboflavin deficiency. In *Advances in Enzyme Regulation*, Vol. 8, G. Weber, ed. Oxford: Pergamon Press, pp. 239–250.

Rivlin, R. S., and R. Hornibrook, 1971a. Thyroid hormone regulation of riboflavin metabolism in newborn rats. *Fed. Proc.* 30:359 (abstract).

Rivlin, R. S., and R. Hornibrook, 1971b. Accelerated development of brain enzymes caused by thyroid hormone. *Program of the Fifty-Third Meeting of the Endocrine Society*, p. 110 (abstract).

Rivlin, R. S., and R. G. Langdon, 1966. Regulation of hepatic FAD levels by thyroid hormone. In *Advances in Enzyme Regulation*, Vol. 4, G. Weber, ed. Oxford: Pergamon Press, pp. 45–58.

Rivlin, R. S., M. Osnos, and R. Hornibrook, 1972. Inhibition of thyroxine-induced tadpole metamorphosis by analogues of riboflavin. International Congress Series No. 256, *Fourth International Congress of Endocrinology*, Washington, D.C., June 18–24, 1972. Amsterdam: Excerpta Medica, p. 245 (abstract).

Rivlin, R. S., and G. Wolf, 1969. Diminished responsiveness to thyroid hormone in riboflavin-deficient rats. *Nature (London)* 223:516–517.

Sokoloff, L., and P. A. Roberts, 1971. Biochemical mechanisms of the action of thyroid hormones in nervous and other tissues. In *Influence of Hormones on the Nervous System*, D. H. Ford, ed. Basal: S. Karger, pp. 213–230.

Sokoloff, L., P. A. Roberts, M. M. Januska, and J. E. Kline, 1968. Mechanisms of stimulation of protein synthesis by thyroid hormones in vivo. *Proc. Nat. Acad. Sci. USA* 60:652–659.

Staal, G. E. J., J. Visser, and C. Veeger, 1969. Purification and properties of glutathione reductase of human erythrocytes, *Biochim. Biophys. Acta* 185:39–48.

Swoboda, B. E., 1969. The relationship between molecular conformation and the binding of flavin-adenine dinucleotide in glucose oxidase. *Biochim. Biophys. Acta* 175:365–379.

Tata, J. R., 1964. Biological action of thyroid hormones at the cellular and molecular levels. In *Actions of Hormones on Molecular Processes*, G. Litwack, and D. Kritchevsky, eds. New York: John Wiley & Sons, pp. 58–131.

Winick, M., 1970. Nutrition and nerve cell growth. *Fed. Proc.* 29:1510–1515.

Wolf, G., and R. S. Rivlin, 1970. Inhibition of thyroid hormone induction of mitochondrial α-glycerophosphate dehydrogenase in riboflavin deficiency. *Endocrinology* 86:1347–1353.

Wolff, E. C., and J. Wolff, 1964. The mechanism of action of the thyroid hormones. In *The Thyroid Gland*, Vol. 1, R. Pitt-Rivers, and W. R. Trotter, eds. London: Butterworths, pp. 237–282.

74 The Chemotactic Response as a Potential Model for Neural Systems

D. E. KOSHLAND, JR.

ABSTRACT Bacterial chemotaxis has been investigated as a potential model for biochemical aspects of neural systems. By developing apparatus to study the quantitative response to bacteria as a population and as individuals, it could be shown that bacteria detect gradients by comparing ratios of concentrations of attractants in the environment. The detection of a gradient apparently involves a rudimentary "memory" mechanism in the sense that the bacteria utilize a time-dependent response that compares past environmental conditions with present ones. This response is in turn mediated by highly specific receptor proteins, of which the ribose binding protein of *Salmonella typhimurium* is one example. There are many analogies at the biochemical and behavioral level between this simple system and higher neural systems, but the extent of the similarities must await further work.

THE RESPONSE OF organisms to chemical stimuli—varying from the odor and taste sensations of man, through the response of insects to pheromones, to the migration of bacteria in gradients of attractants—have certain apparent similarities. For example, the specificities of the responses to a restricted group of chemicals (Moncrieff, 1967) suggest the kind of specificity identified with protein molecules. Moreover, the evidence at all levels indicates that the attractant need not be metabolized in order to provide the stimulus (Weibull, 1960). Since biological patterns tend to recur in nature, the existence of a common biochemical response to stimuli is not unreasonable. However, the fact that nature frequently utilizes alternate pathways to achieve the same final result means that superficial similarities cannot be used to prove biochemical identities. The studies on chemotaxis reported here, therefore, were initiated with the hope that analogies to higher neural processes might exist but with the understanding that such relationships would require evidence and careful analysis.

Chemotaxis in bacteria was discovered in the 1880s by Engelmann (1902) and Pfeffer (1888) who demonstrated that microorganisms were attracted to chemicals and would migrate up a gradient to the position of optimal concentration. Gabricevsky (1900) demonstrated that the bacteria responded positively to some chemicals, negatively to others, and were indifferent to a third group. This phenomenon has been studied by many workers in the subsequent years, most particularly by the discerning studies of Adler and his co-workers on *Escherichia coli* (Adler, 1969). Adler demonstrated that there were two general classes of chemotactic mutants: In one group, called *specific*, mutation eliminated response to a particular chemical, and in a second, called *general*, the bacteria were unable to respond to any chemical attractants (Adler, 1969). The first mutants were presumably identified with the individual receptor molecules for each chemoattractant, the latter with the general apparatus for chemotaxis itself. Recently Hazelbauer and Adler (1971) have studied mutants that indicate that the galactose-binding transport protein, isolated by Boos and Kalckar (Wu et al., 1969), also serves as the receptor in chemotaxis.

Our approach to neural systems was to attempt to correlate the conformational properties of the receptor with the biological response in ways similar to those employed in our laboratory for a number of years on isolated enzyme systems (Koshland and Neet, 1968). It was clear that if such a biochemical approach to chemotaxis were to succeed, added quantitative tools would be needed and the initial studies have been directed to the development of the needed procedures. Three apparatus have been developed, each for a specific purpose. The first, a *migration velocity apparatus*, measures the movement of a mass of bacteria as a statistical average in much the same way that the gross diffusion of a solute in a liquid is described (Dahlquist et al., 1972). The second, which we call a *tracker*, is a device which measures the movement of individual bacteria in a defined spatial gradient (Lovely, Dahlquist, and Koshland, in preparation). The third is a *temporal gradient apparatus*, which allows us to follow the movements of an individual bacterium in a temporal gradient in the absence of a spatial gradient (Macnab and Koshland, 1972). In addition, a receptor for ribose chemotaxis has been isolated. The results allow us to describe the basic features of the mechanism of bacterial chemotaxis and to draw analogies to higher neural systems.

D. E. KOSHLAND, JR. Department of Biochemistry, University of California, Berkeley, California

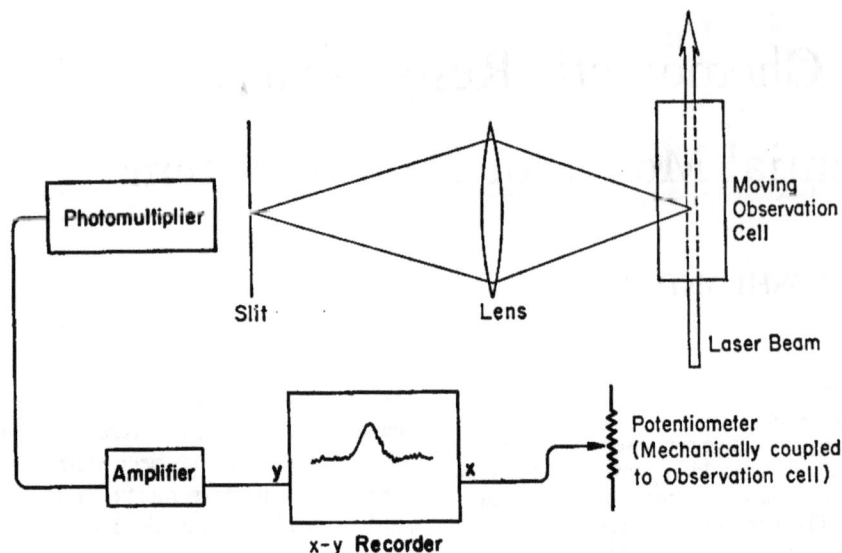

FIGURE 1 Migration velocity apparatus. A schematic representation of the apparatus designed to detect the migration of a bacterial population in a defined gradient.

Migration velocity apparatus and Weber's law

The apparatus designed for measuring the migration of the bacteria as a population was designed by F. Dahlquist and P. Lovely (Dahlquist et al., 1972) and is shown schematically in Figure 1. A linear density gradient of glycerol (0.5 to 3%) is used to stabilize a solution in an observation cell of 10-ml vol, 8-cm high. The bacterial concentration in the cell is determined by monitoring the intensity of light scattered by the bacteria. The light is supplied by an He-Ne laser, which shines up through the bottom of the observation cell. A photomultiplier tube measures the intensity of the laser light scattered at right angles to the beam. At low bacterial concentrations (less than 10^7 bacteria per ml) the intensity of the right-angle scattered light was found to be proportional to the bacterial concentration. The concentration of bacteria at various positions of the cell can be determined by moving the observation cell vertically by means of a screw drive. The cell position is recorded on the x axis and the signal from the photomultiplier is recorded on the y axis of an x–y plotter. The distribution of bacteria in the cell can be scanned in 1 to 3 min and this distribution is then followed as a function of time. By suitable mixing chambers before the introduction of the liquid to the column, various distributions of attractant and/or bacteria can be constructed in the observation cell. In Figure 2 is shown the response of these bacteria to a linear gradient of an attractant, serine, superimposed on an initially uniform distribution of *Salmonella typhimurium*. The gradient runs from zero to 10^{-3} M serine. The bacteria accumulate at the high serine concentration region, but a broad peak is formed in the middle of the serine gradient. This can only be explained if the velocity of the bacteria moving up the gradient depends on the absolute concentration as well as the rate of change of concentration. The gradient dc/dx is constant throughout, so the bacteria cannot be responding solely to the absolute gradient of serine.

An explanation of the complicated response to linear gradients is that the bacteria actually respond to proportional changes in concentration, that is, dc/c. In this case, an exponential gradient

$$\left(\frac{dc/c}{dx} = \frac{d \ln c}{dx} = \text{constant} \right)$$

should elicit a constant bacterial response throughout its length. The result of superimposing such a distribution of serine on an initially uniform bacterial distribution is shown in Figure 3. In this case the bacteria accumulate at the top of the gradient as a well-defined peak. The bacterial concentration on either side of this peak remains fairly constant, however, unlike the response to a linear increase that shows a distinct trough adjacent to the peak. Thus, bacteria are moving through the gradient region at a steady rate. This in turn means that the average velocity of the bacteria is determined by the proportional changes (i.e., ratios) in concentrations. (A trough should and does occur at the bottom of the tube, but it is obscured by scattering of light from the glass bottom.)

Bacterial response to ratios of concentrations can be double checked in another way, as shown in Figure 4. In this case, a steep increase in serine concentration from 2×10^{-3} M to 3×10^{-3} M is imposed over a very short

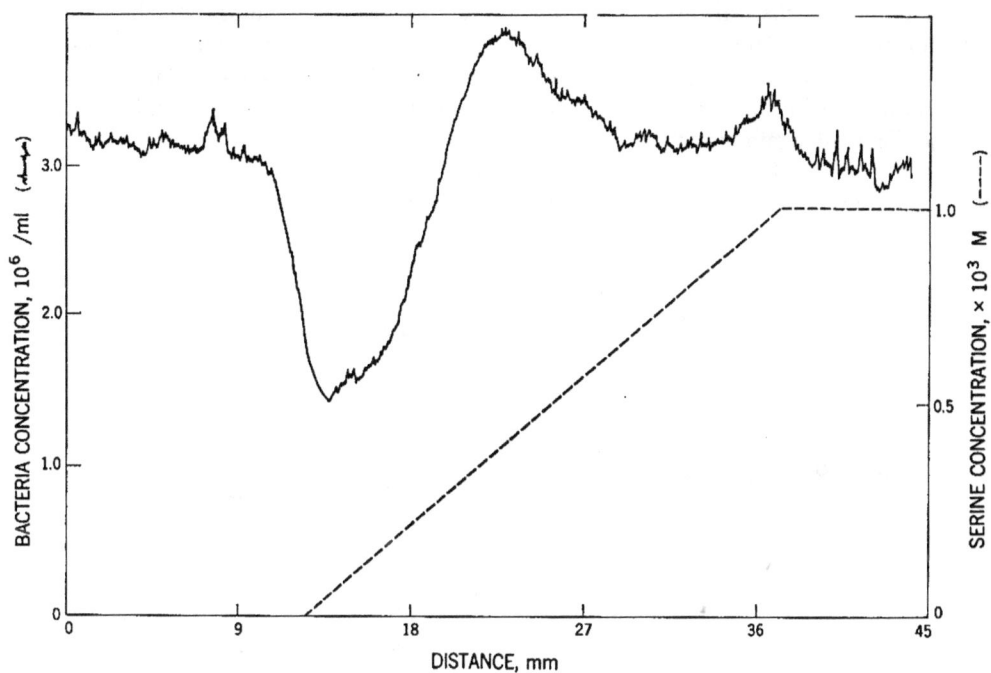

FIGURE 2   The response of *S. typhimurium* to a linear gradient of L-serine (represented by the dashed line). The trace represents the redistribution after 18 min of the bacteria from an initially uniform distribution.

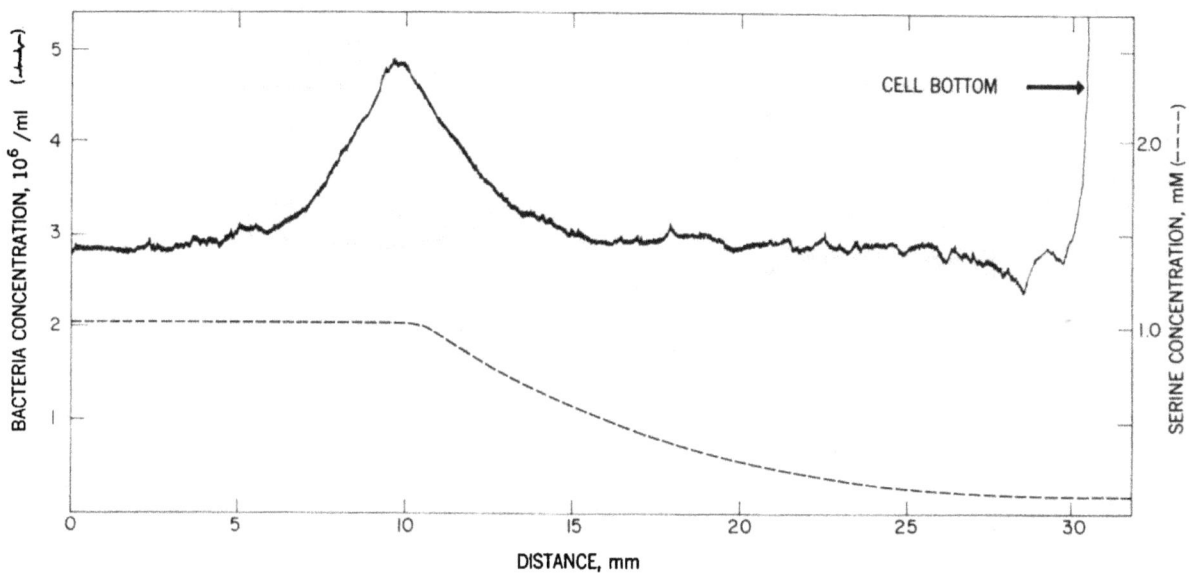

FIGURE 3   The response of *S. typhimurium* to an exponential gradient of L-serine. The plateau concentration of serine employed was 10^{-3} M and the decay distance of the gradient was 6.4 mm. The dashed line represents the initial serine concentration. The trace represents the bacteria redistribution after 15 min.

region of the observation cell on an initially uniform distribution of bacteria. The bacteria at far distances from the gradient, e.g. at the bottom of the cell, do not see any gradient and have no tendency to migrate. Those in the immediate vicinity of the gradient will swim towards the higher serine concentration. The bacteria on the high plateau side of the gradient will again see no gradient and will exhibit no net migration. The net movement of bacteria from low concentrations of serine to high concentrations of serine will therefore produce a trough in the region that bacteria are swimming from and a peak where the bacteria accumulate. If the same *relative gradient* is made in each of the experiments of Figure 4, the response of the bacteria after 20 min is essentially the same. Thus, the ratio across the boundary from 2×10^{-3} M to 3×10^{-3} M is the same as across the boundary from 2×10^{-5} M to 3×10^{-5} M, but the differences in concentrations in these two experiments are altered by a factor of

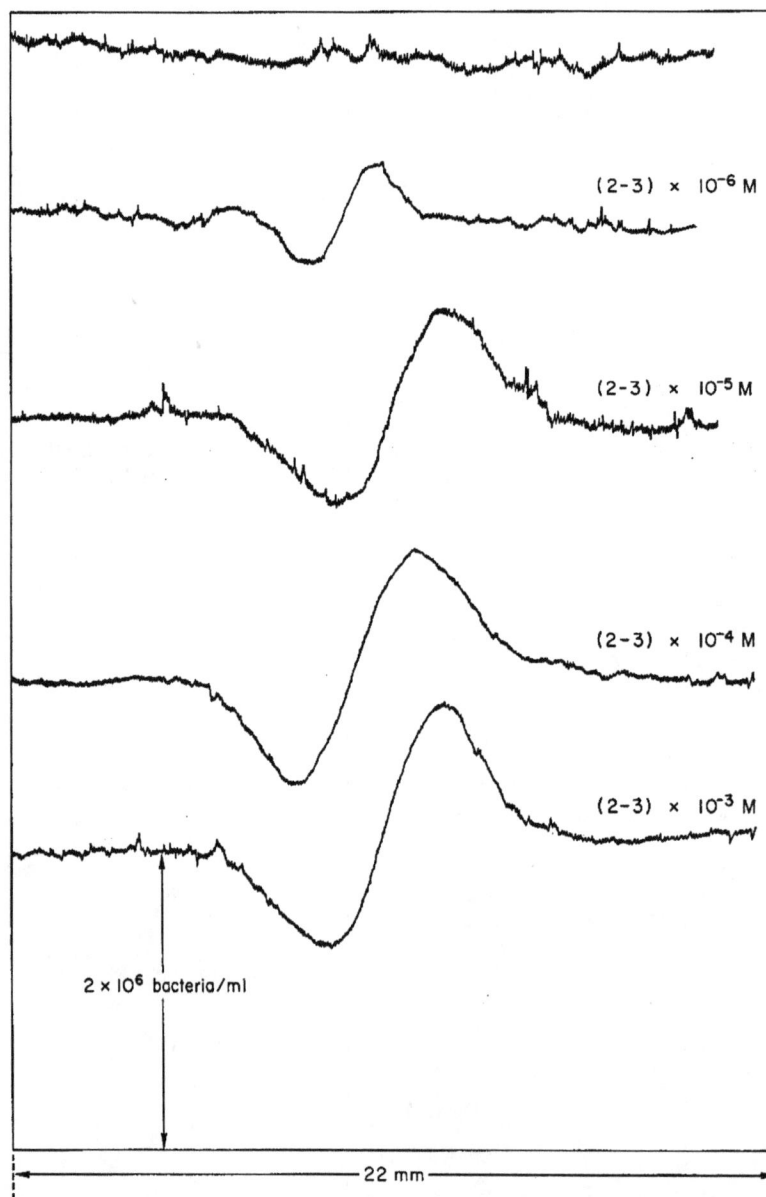

FIGURE 4 Response of bacteria to a constant ratio of attractant concentrations. An initially uniform distribution of *Salmonella* in the colony migration apparatus was exposed to a steep gradient with 2×10^x M attractant on one side and 3×10^x M attractant on the other, where x was varied from -6 to -3. The recordings represent the distribution of bacteria after 15 min. The response is seen to be about the same from 10^{-5} to 10^{-3} M absolute concentration but to drop off somewhat at 10^{-6}.

100. These findings therefore reinforce those of Figure 3, i.e., that the bacteria are responding to ratios not to differences in concentrations.

This leads us to the first of our conclusions, that the bacteria to a very rough approximation follow the Weber-Fechner law (Thompson, 1967). It is of interest that this Weber-Fechner law, which states that the just noticeable increase in a stimulus is proportional to the intensity of the stimulus, has been observed roughly for a wide variety of psychic phenomena, including many responses in higher organisms (Thompson, 1967).

The similarity does not end there. In fact, the obedience to Weber's law is only rough in higher species, and significant deviations occur for the bacteria as well. As discussed above, the bacteria move with uniform velocity through a cell with an exponential gradient extending over a rather limited concentration range. But when this concentration range was varied, the velocities of migration varied so that there is not precise agreement with Weber's law (Dahlquist et al., 1972). The deviations observed were well beyond experimental error and the bacteria deviate from Weber's law by amounts similar to those observed in mammals in psychological tests of phenomena such as the estimation of light intensity, the observations of sounds, the response to pressure, and many other behavioral characteristics (Thompson, 1967).

The "tracker" and the mean free path of bacterial motion

In order to understand the kinetics of chemotaxis and later to study behavioral mutants, we needed a precise description of the motion of an individual bacterium. A device for describing this motion in quantitative terms had been developed by Berg (1971). However, the initial Berg device did not allow the observation of movements of the bacterium in defined stable gradients of attractant. (Since the development of our instrument, Berg has solved the diffusion equation problem. His instrument has advantages in that it follows a bacterium automatically and more accurately than our instrument, but his gradient changes with time and cannot be used for repellents. Our instrument requires manual operation but can be used for observing bacterium in stable defined gradients that may include mixtures of repellents and attractants, two types of attractants, and other complex test systems. Thus, the two instruments complement each other in a very useful way.) The apparatus described in Figure 5 was devised by P. Lovely and F. Dahlquist to solve this problem.

A cuvette, essentially identical to the one in the integration velocity apparatus, is mounted on a microscope stage and bacteria are placed therein in a defined gradient. The long-range objective of a Leitz microscope is focused to see the bacteria in this vessel using dark field optics. The long working distance of the objective (7 mm) allows one to see the bacteria well away from the walls of the vessel. A "joy stick" allows us to activate motors that move the observation cell in the x and z directions and a pedal activates motors which move the cell in the y direction. Using a crosshair in the eyepiece of the microscope and the optical changes in the bacterium, an individual bacterium can be kept in focus by operation of the "joy stick" and the pedal. The motion of the observation cell and hence of the bacterium is recorded on computers and from this a record of the motion in x–y–z coordinates can be reconstructed.

Figure 6 shows a plot of the x, y, and z coordinates of a moving bacterium as a function of time in a zero gradient situation. We can determine the relative up and down motions in various ways, one of which is shown in Table I. Here the distance covered by the bacterium in each 5 sec interval is recorded. The z components of this velocity are then computed to give the velocity in μm/sec.

TABLE I

Average direction velocity of a bacterium when no gradient exists in the medium

Bacterium Tracked	Average Speed in 5 Sec Interval	Average Speed Upward ($+z$)	Average Speed Downward ($-z$)	Ratio
1	19.5 (73)	19.4 (34)	19.7 (29)	0.98
2	27.2 (70)	27.0 (25)	27.3 (45)	0.99
3	20.0 (14)	17.3 (3)	21.8 (11)	0.79
4	22.0 (100)	22.3 (43)	21.8 (57)	1.05
5	21.1 (85)	21.2 (23)	21.0 (62)	1.01

Speeds obtained from determining average speed in 5 sec intervals. Numbers in parentheses refer to number of 5 sec intervals used to determine average.

When the bacteria are moving in a zero gradient situation (i.e., a uniform distribution of attractant or repellent), the average velocity traveling up ($+z$) should be equal to the average traveling down ($-z$), and this is found to be the case. When the bacteria are observed in a gradient, the net velocity upwards exceeds the net velocity downwards and one such set of values is shown in Table II. The average velocity of a bacterium may vary from individual to individual but the average up and down velocities taken over fairly long sampling times are amazingly consistent.

In order to make a strict relationship between the movement of a population and the movement of an individual,

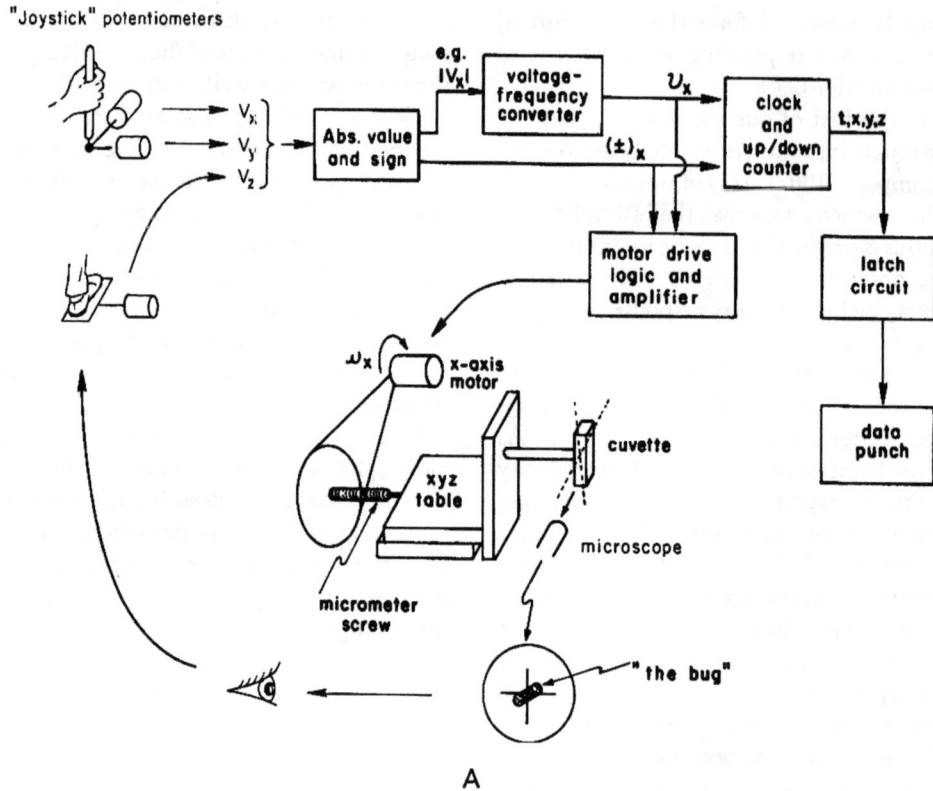

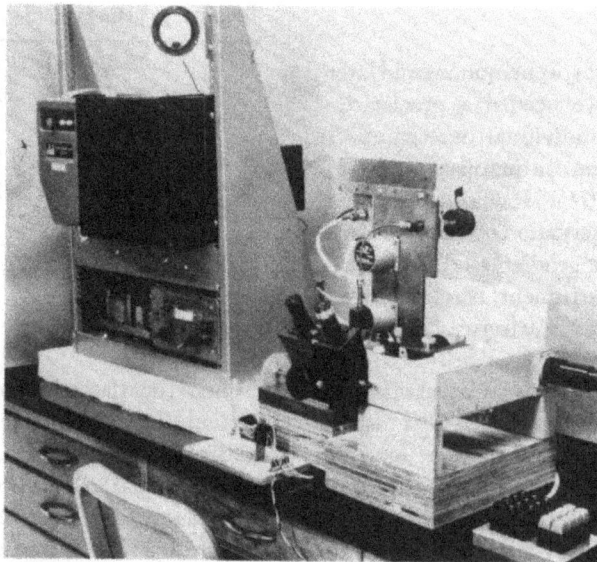

FIGURE 5 (A) Bacterial tracking apparatus. Schematic illustration of device to follow three-dimensional movements of bacteria in the presence and absence of gradients. Observation cell can be filled with bacteria in a defined gradient as described for the migration velocity apparatus. An individual bacterium is kept in focus by movement of this observation cell using the "joy stick" for the x-z directions and the foot pedal for the y direction. Joy stick and pedal activate stepping motors which are connected to punch tape apparatus to record data for calculating coordinates. (B) Photograph of apparatus.

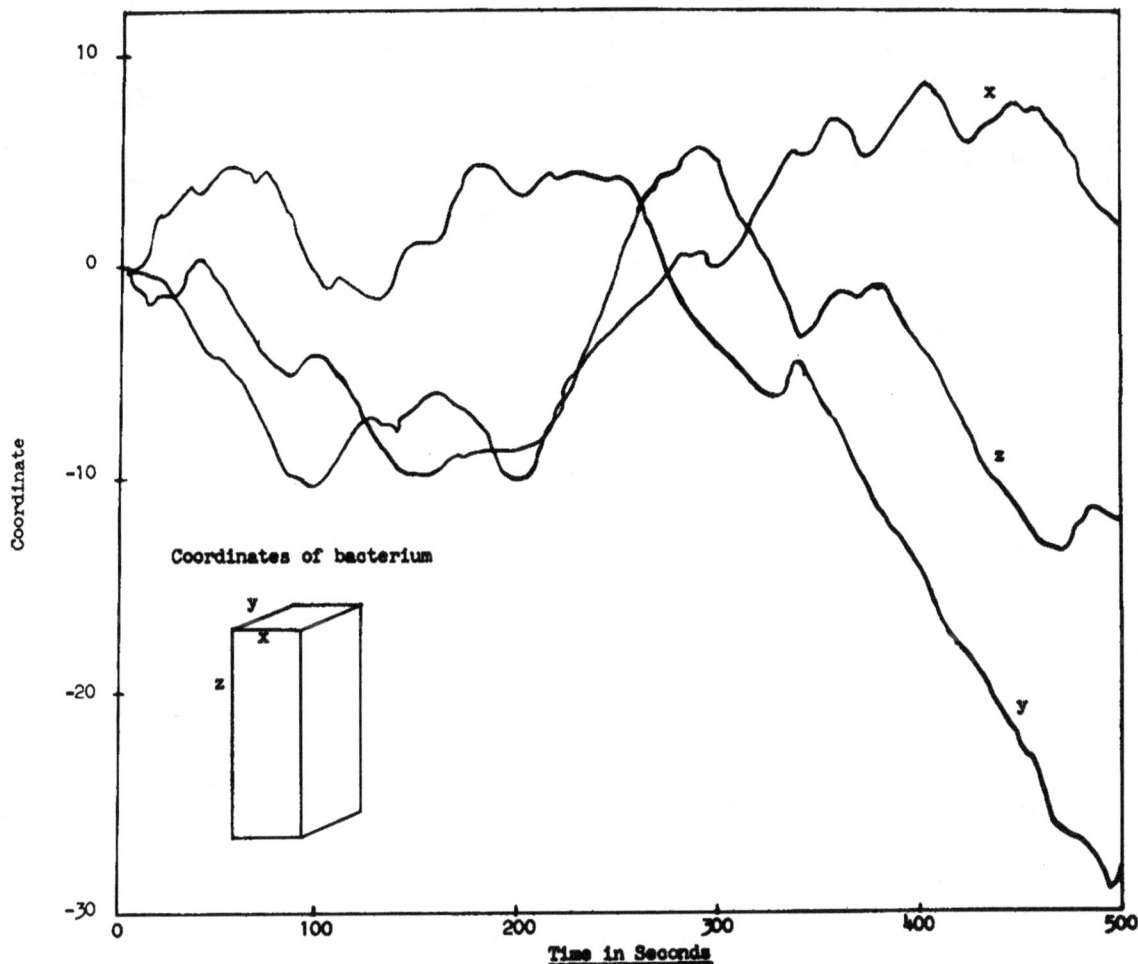

Coordinates of bacterium

FIGURE 6   The movements in space of an individual bacterium followed for 500 sec in the bacterial tracking apparatus.

it is important to have a statistical number of the latter. After tracking a reasonable number of bacteria, the net velocity upwards of a colony of such bacteria was calculated and found to be 2.9 μm/sec. The velocity of the colony as determined by the migration velocity apparatus was 2.8 μm/sec (Dahlquist et al., 1972). This good agreement is pleasing and suggests that both instruments are measuring true characteristics of the bacterial population. Just as in perfect gas theory, the deduction of the collective

TABLE II

Average direction velocity of a bacterium in a gradient of attractant as measured on tracker in serine gradient of 0.15 mm^{-1}

Average % of time traveling up gradient = 60
Average % of time traveling down gradient = 40
   Component of velocity upwards = 11.51 μm sec^{-1}
   Component of velocity downwards = 10.0 μm sec^{-1}
Net average velocity upwards as calculated from tracker =
   0.6 × 11.5 − 0.4 × 10.0 = 2.9 μm/sec
Net average velocity upwards measured in migration velocity
   apparatus = 2.8 μm/sec

properties of a mass can be deduced from the motions of an individual.

What does the tracker indicate about the motions of the individual bacteria? It has previously been observed that the bacteria normally travel for distances in approximately straight lines and tumble at various intervals. This led to the postulation of some type of random-walk mechanism (Armstrong et al., 1967; Keller and Segel, 1971). A variety of such mechanisms can be imagined—some involving modulation of velocity, some of mean free paths, and some of both. The tracker was able to describe the process quantitatively and answer some of these questions.

In the first place, it appears that a given bacterium while it is moving travels through space at an approximately uniform velocity. The increased velocity in the upward direction resulted from less frequent tumbles not from added velocity during the intervals of straight line motion. Thus the observations of the tracker on bacteria in the presence and absence of gradients indicated that a modified random-walk mechanism was a good description of the bacterial movement and that it operated largely, if not completely, through modification of the mean free path and not the velocity of motion.

The temporal gradient apparatus and bacterial "memory"

At this stage we have shown that the bacteria sense a gradient and that they travel up a gradient of attractant by modulating their mean free path. It remains to find how they detect a gradient and how they modulate their mean free path.

In the first place, the difficulties for a bacterium detecting a gradient are very severe. *Salmonella* are approximately 2 μm in length. The drop in concentration of serine in one of the defined gradients described above over a 2 μm length is approximately 1 part in 10^4. A bacterium sensing a gradient by comparing the concentrations of attractant at its head and its tail would therefore be required to contain an analytical apparatus that detects 1 part in 10^4. If one calculates the statistical fluctuations in the more dilute gradient, however, of the individual molecules in the region of the head and the tail of the bacterium, even making very conservative estimates, the fluctuations are approximately 1 part in 10. Thus, the statistical fluctuations would indicate that the bacteria cannot detect a gradient whereas the experimental results indicate that they can. How can one proceed further?

The idea that some time average is involved has been suggested by Delbrück (1972), and time-dependent processes are known in higher species (Thompson, 1967). To test this idea it was necessary to develop an apparatus that could somehow separate temporal processes from spatial processes. The apparatus devised by R. Macnab shown in Figure 7 achieved this purpose (Macnab and Koshland, 1972). Bacteria in a solution containing an initial concentration (c_i) of attractant or repellent are suddenly mixed with a second solution containing the same or different concentrations of the chemical substance. After the mixing is complete, the motions of the bacterium are observed. The observation of the motions of the bacterium are made only when the bacterium is present in a final uniform distribution of chemical, c_f. If the bacterium senses an instanteous spatial gradient, it should behave as it does in a uniform gradient of concentration c_f. If, on the other hand, it has some time-dependent mechanism that allows it to compare the final concentration of its environment (c_f) with the concentration of its near past (c_i) and if the mixing time is fast with respect to this time-sensing mechanism, the bacterium will respond as though it had been swimming in a gradient. Thus, the apparatus is capable of generating a

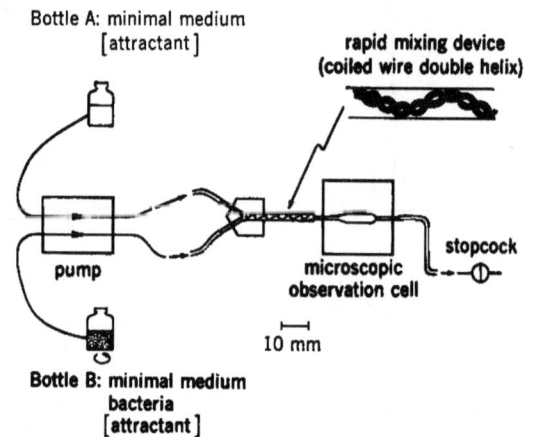

FIGURE 7 Temporal gradient apparatus. Attractant concentrations are: (i) Bottle B, c_i ($\geq$ 0); (ii) bottle A, c_i' ($>$, =, or $< c_i$); (iii) observation cell (as a result of stream mixing) c_f ($>$, =, or $< c_i$). Therefore, bacteria experience a change in concentration from c_i to c_f in a short period of time. They can be subjected to positive, zero, or negative temporal gradients as desired. Gradient is given by $\Delta c/\Delta t$ where $\Delta c = c_f - c_i$ and Δt is mixing time.

temporal gradient, utterly divorced from the spatial gradient. The results obtained are described in detail elsewhere (Macnab and Koshland, 1972), but briefly they are as follows.

If the bacteria are subjected to zero gradient, i.e., $c_i = c_f$ in the temporal gradient apparatus, then motility is *normal*. Normal motility is defined as the motility observed in a wild-type culture in a nongradient situation. The *Salmonella* swam in a fairly coordinated manner, slight changes in direction occurred often, and occasionally a bacterium would tumble and then start swimming in a new direction. A stroboscopic multiple exposure of such behavior is shown in the middle portion of Figure 8. If the bacteria were subject to a positive gradient of attractant, i.e., $c_f > c_i$, supercoordinated swimming was observed, i.e., the bacteria swam for considerably longer distances before tumbling (see upper portion of Figure 8). If on the other hand the bacteria were subjected to a negative gradient of attractant, i.e., $c_f < c_i$, the motion was very uncoordinated, i.e., the bacteria swam only short distances before tumbling and starting out in a new direction (lower portion of Figure 8). These patterns were not the result of the mixing process itself, because bacteria treated in the same way in the absence of a temporal gradient ($c_i = c_f$) showed normal motility. Thus, the bacteria must have a time-dependent mechanism which allows them to remember the concentration of their immediate past (c_i) even though they are presently in a uniform gradient of attractant at a new concentration (c_f). Controls established that the absolute levels of attractant concentration did not affect motility, i.e., the bacteria gave the same normal motility in uniform distributions of attractant at concentrations equal to both c_i and c_f.

The conclusion that a time-dependent process is involved was further supported by the observation of a relaxation process, i.e., the abnormal motility a few seconds after mixing gradually reverts to normal motility during the passage of time. A few *minutes* after plunging into a different concentration $\langle c_i \neq c_f \rangle$ the bacteria that had been subjected to the rapid mixing were indistinguishable from normal bacteria. It, therefore, follows from these experiments that the bacteria are not sensing an immediate spatial gradient but in fact have some device for comparing their previous environment with their present one, i.e., they have some type of primitive *memory* apparatus.

These experiments also answer our previous question about the modulation of the mean free path. It was very difficult in the tracker or by microscopic observation to be sure whether the bacteria migrated by (a) increasing the frequency of tumbling going down the gradient, (2) decreasing their frequency of tumbling going up the gradient, or (3) both. The temporal gradient apparatus indicates that (3) is correct in principle, but the relaxation times indicate (2) may be a better approximation in practise.

Moreover, the apparatus allowed us to test the effect of repellents in a quantitative manner, and it was found (Tsang, Macnab, and Koshland, in preparation) that repellents bear a reciprocal relationship to attractants, i.e., the bacteria tumble more frequently when $c_f > c_i$ and tumble less frequently when $c_f < c_i$.

A good picture of the mechanism of chemotaxis emerges from these experiments. The bacteria do not *sense* an immediate spatial gradient; they, in fact, sense a temporal gradient. In the real world, however, they convert a spatial gradient into a temporal gradient by traveling at uniform velocity through space and integrating or comparing over a time interval. Thus, if they are traveling up a positive gradient of attractant, they move at a constant velocity through increasing concentrations of attractant so they *see* a positive temporal gradient. As a result they tumble less frequently than normal and when they are traveling down such a gradient they tumble more frequently. When traveling in a gradient of a repellent, the responses are reversed, i.e., a positive gradient causes more frequent tumbling, a negative gradient, less frequent.

By integrating over time, they solve two problems that were mentioned previously. In the first place, they eliminate the statistical fluctuation problem by avoiding an instantaneous comparison that would require high accuracy. In the second place, by comparing a concentration in the past with a concentration in the present,

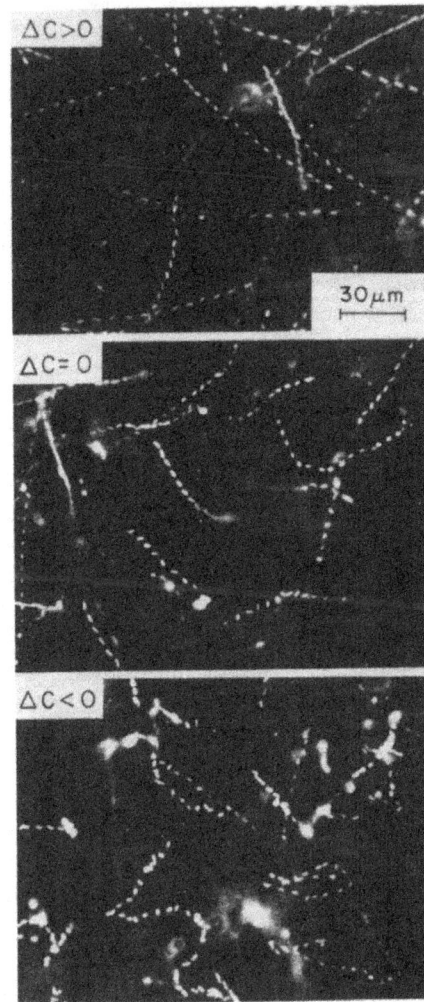

FIGURE 8 Motility tracks of *S. typhimurium,* taken in the time interval 2–7 sec after subjecting bacteria to a sudden (200 msec) change in attractant (serine) concentration in the temporal gradient apparatus. *Upper:* $c_i = 0$, $c_f = 7.6 \times 10^{-4}$ M. Smooth, linear trajectories. *Middle:* $c_i = c_f = 0$ (control). Some changes in direction; bodies often show "wobble" as they travel. Bright spots indicate tumbling or nonmotile bacteria. *Lower:* $c_i = 10^{-3}$ M, $c_f = 2.4 \times 10^{-4}$ M. Poor coordination, frequent tumbles, and erratic changes in direction. [Photomicrographs were taken in dark field with a stroboscopic lamp operating at 5 pulses sec^{-1}. Instantaneous velocity of bacteria in straight line trajectories is of the order of 30 μm sec^{-1}.]

they avoid the problem of their small body size. For example, a bacterium which possesses a *memory* with a decay time of one minute traveling at 30 μm per sec can compare concentrations over an effective distance of 2 mm or roughly 1000 body lengths. The needed analytical accuracy is therefore reduced from 1 part in 10^4 to 1 part in 10.

In paramecium and some higher species, there is a

phenomenon called an *avoidance response* in which an organism reverses direction or flees from a hostile atmosphere. This has been applied to the bacteria in chemotaxis, but our observations in these temporal gradients and in the tracker apparatus would not support such a term for the bacterial behavior. Rather it seems there is a *confusion response*. The bacteria respond to the less favorable direction by increased tumbling, brought about by the apparently uncoordinated motions of their flagella. The loss of coordination with its effect on the mean free path, not a reversal of direction per se, causes the net migration in the opposite direction.

Ribose binding protein

A number of proteins are apparently involved in the transport of metabolites across the bacterial membrane (Pardee, 1968). As mentioned above, one of these, the galactose binding protein of *E. coli* has been identified (Hazelbauer and Adler, 1971) with chemotaxis. Further evidence has been obtained by the isolation of the ribose binding protein of *Salmonella typhimurium*. Using the shock procedure of Heppel (1967) and Anraku (1968), R. Aksamit has purified a ribose binding protein which is a monomer and has a molecular weight of 29,000 (Aksamit and Koshland, 1972).

The specificity of this protein for binding of ribose derivatives is the same as for the chemotactic response (Table III). Both show a very high, if not almost absolute, specificity for ribose. The binding constant of ribose for the pure protein ($K_D = 3.3 \times 10^{-7}$ M) is approximately the same as the midpoint of the chemotactic response curve as determined in the temporal gradient apparatus. The osmotically shocked *Salmonella* bacteria that have lost

their chemotactic response can have it restored by re-addition of the ribose binding protein. Since ribose is a metabolite transported across the membrane of *Salmonella*, it appears that this protein also acts as an agent in the transport of ribose and the chemotaxis toward this attractant. Its similarity to the sulfate binding protein isolated by Langridge, Shinagawa, and Pardee (1970) suggests that its dimensions are similar (72 Å long by 17 Å in diameter), which would allow it to stretch across the membrane if required to do so. The yield of this binding protein indicates that there are about 10^4 receptors per cell of *Salmonella*.

Biochemical mechanism

It remains to consider what biochemical mechanisms are compatible with the observations described above. In order to compare values of a parameter at different times, two component responses to that parameter are required, with different relaxation times. This can be expressed roughly by saying that the fast component response reflects the present value of the parameter, e.g. attractant, while the slow component response reflects the past value. To generate the differential response the component responses must then act in opposing manners on yet another parameter, whose value determines the ultimate response, in this case loss of flagellar coordination. Figure 9 offers one possible scheme of this type. The effector (either the attractant itself or a species generated by it—possibly the attractant-chemoreceptor complex) activates both enzymes 1 and 2 inducing conformational changes, which are fast in enzyme 1 and slow in enzyme 2. These enzymes

TABLE III

Specificity of ribose binding protein and chemotaxis of Salmonella typhimurium

Compound	Chemotaxis Response	Binds to Ribose Binding Protein
Ribose	+ Positive	+
D and L arabinose	No	No
D-xylose	No	No
D-lyxose	No	No
α-D-ribose-1-P	No	No
α-D-methylribofuranose	No	No
1, 4-anhydroribitol	No	No
D-glucose	No	No
D-galactose	No	No
D-mannose	No	No
D-fucose	No	No
L-rhamnose	No	No
α-D-ribose-5-P	No	No
2-deoxy-D-ribose ribitol	No	No

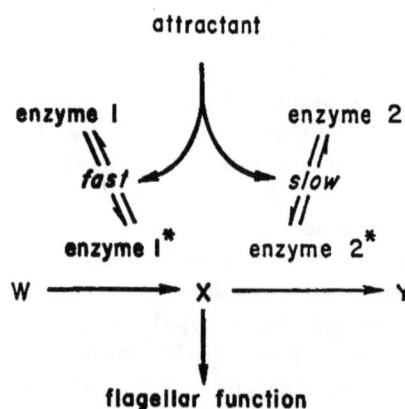

FIGURE 9 Schematic illustration of one possible time-dependent mechanism. Attractant alters conformation of enzymes 1 and 2 to catalytically more active forms, enzyme 1 rapidly and enzyme 2 slowly. The compound X, which controls flagellar function, therefore tends to increase in positive gradients, decrease in negative gradients, remain unchanged in zero gradients.

catalyze the synthesis and degradation respectively of compound X whose pool size must exceed a critical value for the flagella to function in a coordinated manner. In a positive gradient of attractant, enzyme 1 will be more highly activated than enzyme 2, the pool size of X will rise, and tumbling will diminish. In a negative gradient the pool size of X will be depleted and consequently tumbling will increase.

It must be emphasized that this example is only one of a number that can be devised. For example, the enzyme roles could be reversed if high rather than low levels of X were responsible for loss of coordination. The response might be achieved by diffusion or transport processes across the cell membrane rather than by conformational changes in enzymes. Moreover, there may be a series of steps between the binding of the attractant and the effector that controls the temporal process. That the level of an intermediate X is important is further indicated by experiments which show that two gradients of attractant in the same direction are additive; gradients in opposite directions are subtractive.

Relation of chemotaxis to higher neural systems

The signalling processes in a monocellular organism cannot have the complex circuitry of higher species with a central nervous system, but it could quite possibly use similar biochemical pathways and a similar pattern of recording information. The bacterium under consideration is shown in Figure 10. The information received at receptors distributed over the membrane is transmitted to the flagella. The distance the signal must travel is much shorter than in higher species, but the stimulus must be transmitted and must involve a behavioral response. In the case of *Salmonella*, a response to specific chemicals is apparently analogous to the specific responses in higher organisms, e.g. odor in man, and pheromones in insects. The high specificity of the response, e.g. to ribose only, indicates a protein molecule is the receptor and such a molecule has been isolated. The response does not require the metabolism of the attractant as is also true in higher species. An exactly parallel and inverse relationship is seen in repellents. The analogy to pheromones in insects and to taste and odor in mammals is impressive. The bacteria obey Weber's law roughly over short ranges of stimuli and deviate significantly from it over wide ranges, again as seen in higher species.

The bacteria utilize a time-dependent mechanism that can be termed a *memory* in the sense that it allows the bacterium to compare its past with its present. This memory is very short, but it requires a biochemical mechanism which allows an integration over time. Quite

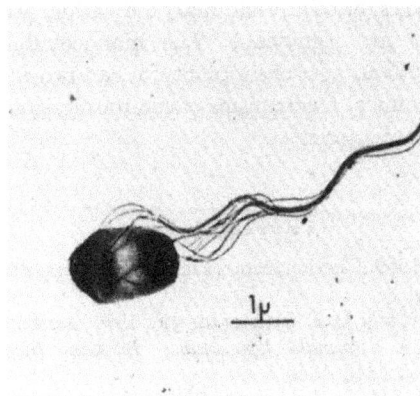

FIGURE 10   An electron microscope picture of a *Salmonella*. The receptors are located in the periplasmic space in the outer membrane. The binding of a chemoattractant generates a signal that is transmitted in some manner to produce a behavioral response in the flagella. (Picture kindly donated by Dr. B. Gerber.)

obviously, this is a long way from the memory of man with its vast storage and retrieval mechanisms. Yet the relation of the bacterial system to higher species may be important, just as the analogy in protein synthesizing pathways between bacteria and higher species is close but not identical.

The mechanism proposed in Figure 9 indicates that the level of some chemicals is critical for the signal to the flagella. Moreover the inputs to this level from a variety of attractants and repellents act as a summation process. Such levels could logically be related to equivalent levels in a neuron. In that case the state of polarization depends on additive and subtractive relationships of stimuli from chemicals, dendrites, and hormones. Moreover the signal in the bacteria is transmitted from the receptor to the flagella just as a signal in higher species must be transmitted from a receptor to the motor apparatus. The distances are greater in the latter case but again the chemistry may have common features.

Finally, if new interneuron connections are to be initiated or reenforced by the synthesis of new proteins or are to be deleted by hydrolysis of old proteins and decreased protein synthesis, some change in chemical level is indicated. Small molecules such as cyclic AMP, inducers or corepressors are required to initiate protein synthesis or inhibit protein breakdown. It is logical therefore that a change in the level of some compound X could itself trigger other more permanent chemical changes as well as being involved with the firing of an individual neuron. Learning and memory might therefore be products of a common biochemical event.

The behavior patterns of the single-cell bacteria will obviously be simpler than the more complex processes in higher species, but the preliminary indications are that the similarities are significant. The monocellular system offers the advantages of simplicity; it can provide insight into biochemical mechanisms of communication that are common to all species.

REFERENCES

ADLER, J., 1969. Chemoreceptors in bacteria. *Science* 166:1588–1597.

AKSAMIT, R., and D. E. KOSHLAND, JR., 1972. A ribose binding protein of *Salmonella typhimurium*. *Biochem. Biophys. Res. Commun.* 48:1348–1353.

ANRAKU, Y., 1968. Transport of sugars and amino acids in bacteria. I. Purification and specificity of the galactose- and leucine-binding proteins. *J. Biol. Chem.* 243:3116–3122.

ARMSTRONG, J. B., J. ADLER, and M. A. DAHL, 1967. Non-chemotactic mutants of *Escherichia coli*. *J. Bacteriol.* 93:390–398.

BERG, H. C., 1971. How to track bacteria. *Rev. Sci. Instrum.* 42:868–871.

DAHLQUIST, F. W., P. LOVELY, and D. E. KOSHLAND, JR., 1972. Quantitative analysis of bacterial migration in chemotaxis. *Nature New Biology* 236:120–123.

DELBRÜCK, M., 1972. Signal transducers: *Terra incognita* of molecular biology. *Angew. Chem. (Eng.)* 11:1–6.

ENGELMANN, T. W., 1902. Die Erscheinungsweise der Sauerstoffaus scheidung chromophyl haltiger Zellen im Licht bei Anwendung der Bakterienmethode. *Pflüger Arch. Ges. Physiol.* 57:375–390.

GABRICEVSKY, G. N., 1900. Uber Aktive Beweglichkeit der Bakterien. *Z. Ges. Hyg.* 35:104–122.

HAZELBAUER, G. L., and J. ADLER, 1971. Role of galactose binding protein in chemotaxis of *Escherichia coli* toward galactose. *Nature New Biology* 230:101–104.

HEPPEL, L. A., 1967. Selective release of enzymes from bacteria. *Science* 156:1451–1455.

KELLER, E. F., and L. A. SEGEL, 1971. Model for chemotaxis. *J. Theor. Biol.* 30:225–234.

KOSHLAND, D. E., JR., and K. E. NEET, 1968. The catalytic and regulatory properties of enzymes. *Ann. Rev. Biochem.* 37:359–410.

LANGRIDGE, R., H. SHINAGAWA, and A. B. PARDEE, 1970. Sulfate-binding protein from *Salmonella typhimurium*: Physical properties. *Science* 169:59–61.

MACNAB, R. M., and D. E. KOSHLAND, JR., 1972. The gradient-sensing mechanism in bacterial chemotaxis. *Proc. Nat. Acad. Sci. USA* 69:2509–2512.

MONCRIEFF, R. W., 1967. *The Chemical Senses*. London: Leonard Hill.

PARDEE, A. B., 1968. Membrane transport proteins. *Science* 162:632–637.

PFEFFER, W., 1888. *Untersuch Botan. Inst. Tubingen* 2:582–661.

THOMPSON, R. F., 1967. *Foundations of Physiological Psychology*. New York: Harper and Row.

WEIBULL, C., 1960. Movement. In *The Bacteria*. Vol. I. I. C. Gunsalus and R. Y. Stanier, ed. New York: Academic Press, pp. 153–202.

WU, H. C. P., W. BOOS, and H. M. KALCKAR, 1969. Role of the galactose transport system in the retention of intracellular galactose in *Escherichia coli*. *J. Mol. Biol.* 41:109–120.

75 Regulation of Allosteric Enzymes in Glutamine Metabolism

STANLEY PRUSINER

ABSTRACT   The intracellular levels of many enzymes are under precise control by specific metabolite inducers and corepressors and by cyclic AMP. In addition, the catalytic activity of many enzymes is modulated both allosterically and isosterically by specific metabolite ligands. The enzymes involved with glutamine metabolism illustrate several of the principles of enzyme regulation. Since the synthesis and degradation of glutamine lies at a crossroads where carbohydrate and nitrogen metabolism intersect, and since glutamine is the amide nitrogen donor for the biosynthesis of amino acids, nucleotides, amino sugars and cofactors, it is not unexpected that many enzymes and metabolites influence the intracellular concentration of glutamine. Indeed, diverse and rigorous control mechanisms have been found to participate in the regulation of glutamine metabolism in microorganisms. A knowledge of these control mechanisms may be of value in understanding both the physiological and pathological metabolism of nitrogen in the nervous system.

IN BIOLOGICAL organisms almost all of the chemical reactions that occur are catalyzed by specific enzymes. The cellular concentration of particular enzymes and the modulated activity of these enzymes are complex processes as described in two preceding chapters by Drs. Schimke and Koshland.

This communication gives examples of the complex and elegant enzymatic machinery that has evolved to regulate the intracellular levels of glutamate and glutamine in microorganisms (Prusiner and Stadtman, 1973). A discussion of the enzymatic regulation of glutamate and glutamine metabolism is especially relevant to neurobiology, because glutamate, glutamine, aspartate, and γ-aminobutyric acid account for more than 70% of the nonprotein amino nitrogen in nervous tissue (Himwich and Agrawal, 1969). Of these amino acids, glutamate predominates and is present in a concentration of at least 10 mM while glutamine is present *at* 4 mM.

The neuroscience literature on glutamine and glutamate metabolism is immense, because these amino acids have been studied extensively with regard to synaptic transmission (Johnson, 1972; Bloom, 1972), compart-

mentation of the brain (Waelsch, 1951; Salganicoff and DeRobertis, 1965; Van Den Berg, 1970; Berl and Clarke, 1970; Rose, 1970), epilepsy (Sourkes, 1962), mental retardation (Sourkes, 1962), schizophrenia (Roberts, 1972), hepatic failure (Walker and Schenker, 1970; Williams et al., 1972) and hyperammonemia (Shih and Efron, 1972; Ghadimi, 1972). No attempt to review these studies is made here.

In Figure 1, the assimilation of NH_4^+ into glutamate and glutamine and the possible fates of the ammonia nitrogen are illustrated. The interconversion of glutamate and glutamine lie at a crossroads where carbohydrate and nitrogenous metabolism intersect. The amino nitrogen of glutamate may be transferred to keto-acids by several transaminases, while the carbon skeleton of glutamate may be consumed in the tricarboxylic acid cycle. Glutamine may donate its amide nitrogen to a variety of reactions which participate in the biosynthesis of amino acids, amino sugars, nucleotides, and cofactors (Prusiner and Stadtman, 1973).

Enzymatic regulation in two microorganisms

The intricate mechanisms of regulation of the enzymes of glutamate and glutamine metabolism are best understood in bacteria, but they may serve as a model for similar types of control in mammalian cells. Regulation of glutamate and glutamine levels in microorganisms is accomplished in a variety of different ways. A comparison of six enzymes concerned with the metabolism of glutamate and glutamine in *Escherichia coli* and *Bacillus subtilis* reveals that these organisms contain different enzymatic machinery (Table I). *E. coli* and *B. subtilis* both contain glutamine synthetase that catalyzes the synthesis of glutamine from glutamate, ATP, and ammonia:

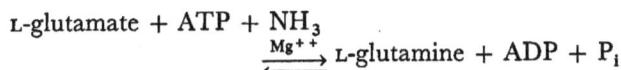

$$\text{L-glutamate} + \text{ATP} + \text{NH}_3 \underset{\longleftarrow}{\overset{\text{Mg}^{++}}{\longrightarrow}} \text{L-glutamine} + \text{ADP} + \text{P}_i$$

The reaction requires a divalent cation, which is probably Mg^{++} in the cell. *B. subtilis* possesses a second enzyme specifically for the synthesis of glutamine to be incorporated into protein (Wilcox, 1969). The reaction involves the

STANLEY PRUSINER   National Heart and Lung Institute, National Institutes of Health, Laboratory of Biochemistry, Bethesda, Maryland

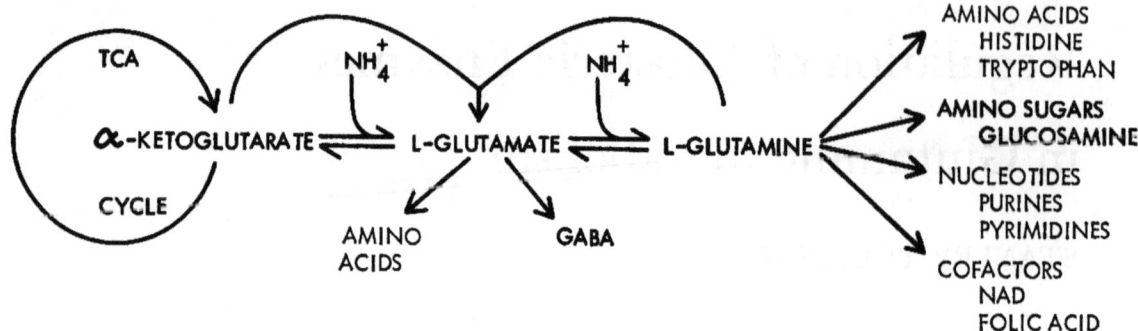

FIGURE 1   The assimilation of NH_4^+ into glutamate and glutamine and the fates of ammonia nitrogen.

TABLE I

Comparison of enzymes involved in the metabolism of glutamate and glutamine in microorganisms

Enzyme	Microorganism		References
	E. coli	*B. subtilis*	
1. Glutamine synthetase	+	+	(Woolfolk and Stadtman, 1964; Deuel et al., 1970)
2. Glutaminyl t-RNA amidotransferase	–	+	(Peterkofsky, 1972; Wilcox, 1969)
3. Glutamate synthase	+	+	(Meers et al., 1970; Elmerich and Aubert, 1971)
4. Glutamate dehydrogenase	+		(Elmerich and Aubert, 1971)
5. Glutaminase A	+		(Hartman, 1968)
6. Glutaminase B	+		(Prusiner and Stadtman, 1971)

+ = present
– = not found

transfer of the amide nitrogen of glutamine or asparagine to glutamyl-t-RNA to form glutaminyl t-RNA. The enzyme has not been detected in *E. coli* (Peterkofsky, 1972).

Both organisms also have the enzyme, glutamate synthase, which was recently discovered by Tempest and coworkers (Meers et al., 1970). The enzyme is an iron sulfide flavoprotein which catalyzes the conversion of α-ketoglutarate and glutamine to two molecules of glutamate in the presence of TPNH (Miller and Stadtman, 1972):

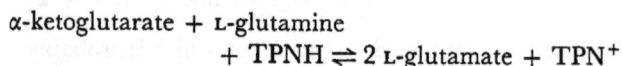

α-ketoglutarate + L-glutamine
$$+ \ TPNH \rightleftharpoons 2 \ \text{L-glutamate} + TPN^+$$

A deficiency of this enzyme in *B. subtilis* results in glutamate auxotrophy (Elmerich and Aubert, 1971). In *E. coli*, glutamate auxotrophy requires a deficiency of both glutamate synthetase and glutamate dehydrogenase (Berberich, 1972).

The glutamate dehydrogenase of *E. coli* is a freely reversible enzyme that catalyzes the conversion of glutamate to α-ketoglutarate and ammonia:

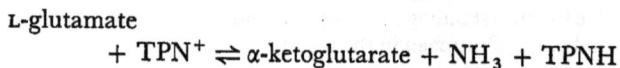

L-glutamate
$$+ \ TPN^+ \rightleftharpoons \text{α-ketoglutarate} + NH_3 + TPNH$$

Also in *E. coli*, there are two glutaminases, A and B, that catalyze the hydrolytic deamidation of L-glutamine to L-glutamate + NH_3 (Hartman, 1968; Prusiner and Stadtman, 1971):

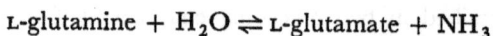

$$\text{L-glutamine} + H_2O \rightleftharpoons \text{L-glutamate} + NH_3$$

These isoenzymes are readily distinguished and separable since glutaminase A is active at pH 5 while B is active at pH 7. No information about glutaminases in *B. subtilis* is available at present.

The differences in enzymatic machinery between the two microorganisms, *E. coli* and *B. subtilis*, in the regulation of glutamine metabolism emphasize the potential variability in enzymatic regulation of metabolism that may exist among different cell types, especially in a mammalian system, such as the brain (Rose, 1970).

Control of enzyme levels

Many studies have demonstrated that microorganisms, like some mammalian cells, have the ability to alter intracellular enzyme levels in response to changes in nutritional conditions. The effect of ammonia on the levels of 5 enzymes concerned with glutamate and glutamine metabolism in *E. coli* are summarized in Table II. Glutamine synthetase levels increased when growth of *E. coli* was limited by the availability of ammonia salts (Woolfolk and Stadtman, 1964; Prusiner et al., 1972). Glutamate synthetase levels also increased when the culture media contained low concentrations of NH_4^+. The response in *Aerobacter aerogenes* was much greater than in *E. coli* (Meers et al., 1970; Miller and Stadtman, 1972). The levels of glutamic dehydrogenase and glutaminase A both decreased with the growth of *E. coli* on low concentrations of NH_4^+ (Pateman, 1969; Prusiner et al., 1972). The ammonia concentration in the growth media did not alter the level of glutaminase B (Prusiner et al., 1972).

TABLE II
The effect of ammonia on the levels of enzymes concerned with the metabolism of glutamate and glutamine in E. coli

Enzyme	Enzyme Levels with Growth on	
	Low NH_4Cl	High NH_4Cl
1. Glutamine synthetase	↑	↓
2. Glutamate synthase	↑	↓
3. Glutamate dehydrogenase	↓	↑
4. Glutaminase A	↓	↑
5. Glutaminase B	↔	↔

↑ increased
↓ decreased
↔ no change

The levels of many enzymes in bacteria are altered by adenosine 3′:5′-cyclic monophosphate (Pastan and Perlman, 1970). Recent studies have disclosed that exogenous cAMP increases the levels of glutamine synthetase and glutamic dehydrogenase and decreases the levels of glutamate synthase and glutaminase A (Prusiner et al., 1972). As shown in Figure 2, the addition of 5 mM cAMP to a logarithmically growing culture of *E. coli* K12 deficient in adenyl cyclase resulted in a doubling of the growth rate and a doubling of the levels of glutamate dehydrogenase and glutamine synthetase. The levels of glutaminase A and glutamate synthase decreased more than 50% in one generation. The level of glutaminase B was not influenced by cAMP. Growth on glycerol, which has been shown to elevate the intracellular level of cAMP in *E. coli*, mimicked the alterations brought about by exogenous cAMP. The effects of cAMP were abolished by chloramphenicol or a deficiency of cAMP receptor protein (Pastan and Perlman, 1970). In mammals, reciprocal effects of cAMP on the enzymes of glycogen metabolism have been observed. These effects involve the covalent chemical modification of pre-existing glycogen phosphorylase and glycogen synthetase by a protein kinase (Soderling et al., 1970). In contrast, the changes in enzyme levels described above appear to involve altered protein synthesis and/or degradation.

In summary, at least three mechanisms participate in the control of enzyme levels in *E. coli*: (1) generalized or

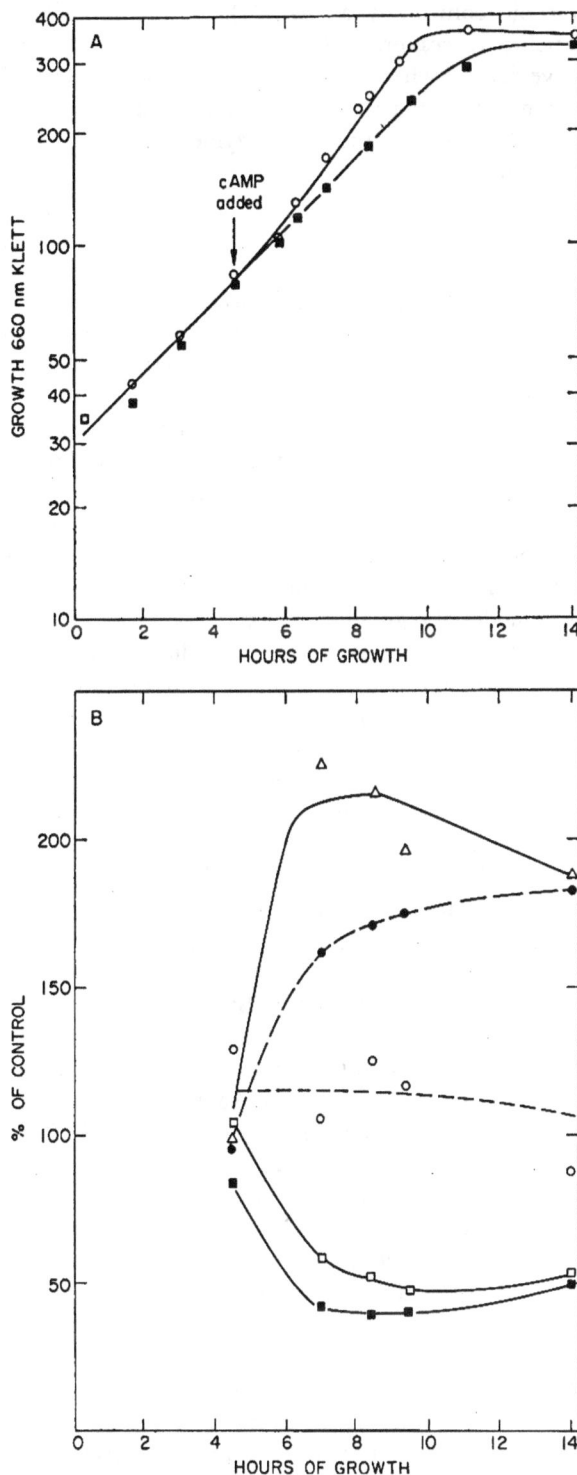

FIGURE 2 Effect of cAMP on *E. coli* K12–5336 growth rate and enzyme levels. (A) Growth of *E. coli* deficient in adenylate cyclase (■——■) 5mM cAMP added at *arrow* (O——O). (B) Changes in specific activities (units/mg) of glutaminase A (■——■), glutamate synthase (□——□), glutamate dehydrogenase (●——●) glutamine synthetase (△——△) and glutaminase B (O——O) at various times after addition of cAMP (for details, see Prusiner et al., 1972).

pleiotropic control by cAMP, (2) specific control by metabolite repression and/or induction, and (3) constitutive control where enzyme levels are independent of nutritional conditions. These control mechanisms may operate through alterations in enzyme synthesis and/or degradation.

Regulation of enzyme activity

In addition to the control mechanisms that regulate the levels of the five enzymes noted above, at least three other types of control act to modulate the activity of these enzymes: (1) allosteric or isosteric feedback inhibition by specific end products or energy metabolites, (2) covalent modification of glutamine synthetase by adenylylation, and (3) divalent cation modulation of enzyme activity directly or through chelation with ATP. Studies on glutamine synthetase and glutaminase B from *E. coli* and on glutamine synthetase from *B. subtilis* illustrate these various modes of regulation of enzyme activity.

Glutamine synthetase from *E. coli* has a molecular weight of 600,000 with 12 subunits of 50,000 molecular weight each arranged in a double layer hexagon (Figure 3). The enzyme is an acidic protein and is subject to feedback inhibition by 8 biosynthetic end products that include histidine, tryptophan, CTP, AMP, glucosamine 6-P, carbamyl phosphate, alanine, and glycine (Stadtman et al., 1968). The sensitivity to feedback inhibitors is dramatically changed by adenylylation of the enzyme (Figure 4). Adenylylation of glutamine synthetase is catalyzed by the enzyme complex P_IP_{II} designated adenylyltransferase in Figure 4 (Stadtman, 1971). The reaction results in the covalent attachment of 1 AMP to 1 specific tyrosine residue in each subunit via a phosphodiester bond. Removal of the AMP involves a pyrophosphorolysis catalyzed by the uridylylated P_IP_{II} enzyme complex (Brown et al., 1971). The adenylylation-deadenylylation process is modulated by divalent cations, α-ketoglutarate, and glutamine. The stimulation of adenylylation by glutamine appears to be an alternate mode of product inhibition since the covalent modification of glutamine synthetase results in a marked decrease in Mg^{++} dependent activity. Mg^{++} is the predominant intracellular divalent cation and probably supports the glutamine synthetase reaction in vivo. Adenylylation lowers the pH optimum of the enzyme and increases the Mn^{++} supported activity. Divalent cations are bound to the enzyme directly and are chelated by ATP. There are 389 distinct forms of glutamine synthetase due to adenylylation of individual subunits (Stadtman, 1971), and the hetereotropic interactions between subunits allow for extensive modulation of enzymatic catalysis.

The regulation of glutamine synthetase from *B. subtilis*

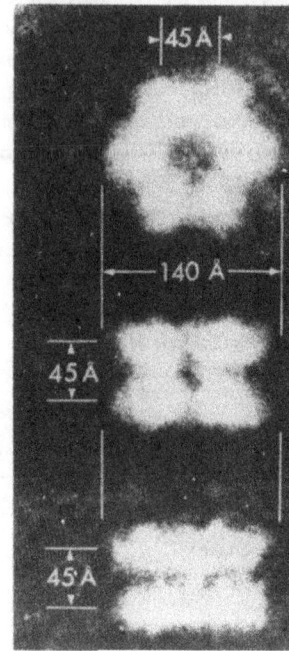

FIGURE 3 Five superimposed electron microscopic images of glutamine synthetase from *E. coli* in three orientations. The upper portion shows a picture of the molecule as it is seen when resting on a face. The center and bottom pictures are views of the molecule as seen on edge when looking exactly down a diameter between subunits or in general as two lines (from Valentine et al., 1968).

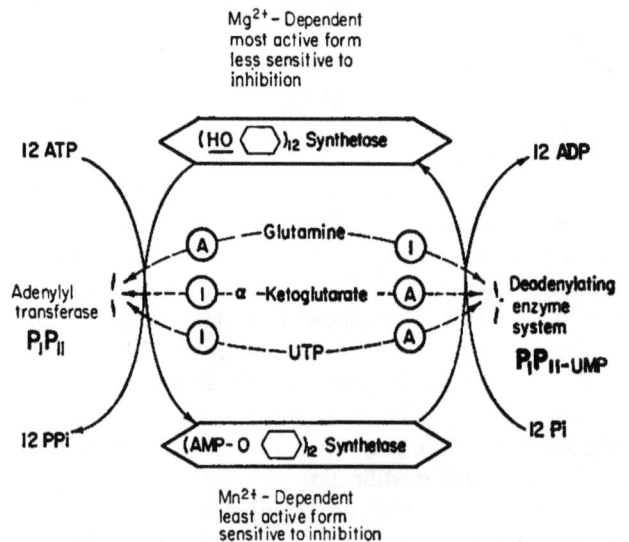

FIGURE 4 Metabolite regulation of adenylylation and deadenylylation reactions which alter divalent cation specificity, catalytic activity, and feedback inhibition of glutamine synthetase from *E. coli* (adapted from Stadtman, 1971).

is distinctly different from *E. coli*, but the structure of the enzyme is similar. The enzyme from *B. subtilis* has a molecular weight of ~600,000 and is composed of 12 identical subunits arranged in a double-layer hexagon. The enzyme requires divalent cations for activity and is subject to feedback inhibition by the same biosynthetic end products, as described for *E. coli*. A complex system of covalent modification involving adenylylation-deadenylylation to regulate the activity of glutamine synthetase under various conditions of nitrogen metabolism does not exist in *B. subtilis* (Gancedo and Holzer, 1968; Deuel et al., 1970). Instead, the organism possesses a glutamine synthetase which is directly susceptible to feedback inhibition by its product, glutamine (Deuel and Prusiner, 1973). As described above, glutamine synthetase from *E. coli* is not inhibited by glutamine but by glutamine-stimulated adenylylation of the enzyme that results in a decrease in the magnesium supported biosynthetic activity. In addition, it is of interest to compare the inhibition by AMP of glutamine synthetase from both organisms, because AMP is not only a biosynthetic end product but also an indicator of cellular energy metabolism. As shown in Figure 5 the *E. coli* enzyme in the unadenylylated form is only moderately inhibited by AMP, but following glutamine-stimulated adenylylation there is a substantial increase in the susceptibility of the enzyme to inhibition by AMP (Ginsburg, 1969; Stadtman, 1971). This same phenomena is even more striking in *B. subtilis*, which does not use adenylylation. Here AMP is not a potent inhibitor; however, the presence of noninhibitory concentrations of glutamine does convert AMP to a powerful inhibitor (Deuel and Prusiner, 1973). This pattern of regulation is designated synergistic feedback inhibition when the inhibition by two ligands is

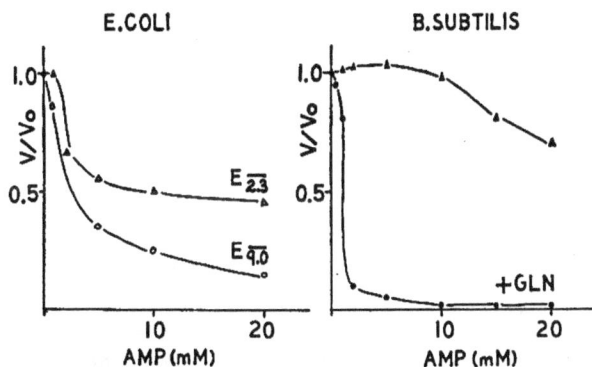

FIGURE 5 Inhibition of glutamine synthetases by AMP. Enzyme activities were measured using the biosynthetic reaction with saturating concentrations of substrates and Mg^{++}. (A) *E. coli* glutamine synthetase activities at two states of adenylylation $E_{\overline{2.3}}$ and $E_{\overline{9.0}}$ (adapted from Ginsburg, 1969). (B) *B. subtilis* glutamine synthetase activities in the presence and absence of 2.5 mM L-glutamine (adapted from Deuel and Prusiner, 1973).

much greater than the sum of the inhibition produced by each ligand independently (Stadtman, 1970). Synergistic effects have been observed with several other enzymes: Phosphoribosyl pyrophosphate amidotransferase from chicken liver (Caskey et al., 1964), aspartokinase from *E. coli* (Truffa-Bachi and Cohen, 1966) and glutamine synthetase from *Bacillus lichenformis* (Hubbard and Stadtman, 1967).

Like the glutamine synthetase of *E. coli*, the enzyme of *B. subtilis* is also able to use Mn^{++} in place of Mg^{++}. In most biological organisms, the intracellular Mg^{++} concentration is 10^2 to 10^4 times greater than Mn^{++} (Silver et al., 1970) but in sporulating bacteria such as *B. subtilis*, the Mn^{++} is accumulated in large quantities during sporulation. The Mn^{++} is obligatory for sporulation and the Mn^{++} content of spores is equal to that of Mg^{++} (Murrell, 1969). The potential modulation of enzyme activity by the interaction of these divalent cations with glutamine synthetase during sporulation and germination may be significant, because glutamine, but not glutamate, represses sporulation (Elmerich and Aubert, 1972).

The action of glutamine synthetase is directly opposed by the enzyme glutaminase. In *E. coli*, there are two glutaminases, as described above, but only glutaminase B is active in the pH range where glutamine synthetase also exhibits activity. In the absence of appropriate controls, the coupling of glutamine synthetase with glutaminase B would form a "futile cycle" of amide synthesis and degradation that would lead to a depletion of cellular energy stores. Several of these potential "futile cycles" have been described (Stadtman, 1970), and they are usually situated at control points in amphibolic pathways, where the anabolic enzyme is regulated by specific biosynthetic end products and the catabolic enzyme by energy metabolites (Sanwal, 1970).

In contrast to glutamine synthetase, the synthesis of glutaminase B is under constitutive control and the enzyme is present in minute quantities (<0.01% of cellular protein). Glutaminase B has a molecular weight of ~90,000, and preliminary studies show that it is probably composed of 3 or 4 subunits. Like many regulatory enzymes, glutaminase B is cold labile, which means that it is reversibly inactivated upon exposure to 4°C and reactivated when heated at 23°C. Ligands such as borate and L-glutamate protect against inactivation by cold. To date, more than 30 enzymes have been found which exhibit this phenomena of cold lability. The molecular basis of cold lability is thought to involve the weakening of hydrophobic bonds as the temperature is lowered (Scheraga et al., 1962).

The activity of glutaminase B can also be altered by preincubation with adenine nucleotides at 4°C. Preincubation with ATP or ADP results in a biphasic curve with activation at concentrations below 1 mM followed by inhibition at higher concentrations (Figure 6). Here AMP is an activator. The presence of adenine nucleotides in the assay is without effect. Maximum inhibition by 10 mM ATP occurred upon preincubation at 4°C for 30 min. The inhibition was reversible upon gel filtration or dialysis if activating ligands were present. The results suggest that glutaminase B exists in a conformation susceptible to ATP inhibition at 4°C and that ATP induces a conformational change that can only be reversed in the presence of activating ligands.

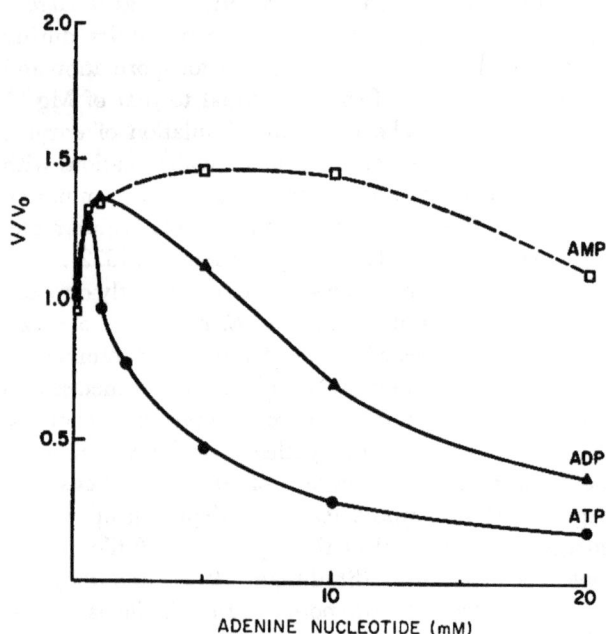

FIGURE 6 Effects of adenine nucleotides on glutamine B activity from *E. coli*. The enzyme was preincubated with the appropriate concentration of nucleotide at 4°C for 30 min prior to assay (for details see Prusiner and Stadtman, 1971).

The regulation of glutaminase B activity by ATP may be modified by AMP that produces synergistic inhibition with ATP. The kinetics of these studies predict at least two nucleotide binding sites on the enzyme. Divalent cations also modify the inhibition due to ATP by directly activating glutaminase B and by chelation with ATP. It is noteworthy that enzymes such as glutaminase B and fumarase (Penner and Cohen, 1969), which are susceptible to ATP inhibition, are not inhibited when ATP is complexed with divalent cations. In contrast, enzymes such as glutamine synthetase and hexokinase, which use ATP as a substrate, require ATP to be complexed with divalent cations for activity. These studies illustrate the potential flexibility of multimeric proteins to respond to a variety of metabolite information.

Measurements of metabolite levels in *E. coli* by Schutt and Holzer (1972) provide additional support for the proposed roles and cellular regulation of glutamine synthetase and glutaminase B. *E. coli* were grown on a glucose-proline minimal media. At time 0, the cells were given 10 mM NH_4Cl, and as shown in Figure 7, the NH_4^+ was immediately assimilated into glutamine while the concentration of ATP dropped 90%. Concomitantly, the level of glutamate decreased, and activity of glutamine synthetase rapidly diminished due to glutamine-stimulated adenylylation, which resulted in a cessation of glutamine synthesis. The depletion of ATP stores threatened cellular survival and presumably relieved the inhibition of glutaminase B by ATP. Glutaminase B could then function to deamidate glutamine, thus making more glutamate available for energy generation in the tricarboxylic acid cycle. This would then lead to a replenishment of ATP stores. The reduction of cellular glutamine stores by glutaminase B would also be advantageous for conserving energy stores, since numerous biosynthetic reactions which utilize ATP would then be turned off.

Figure 8 summarizes the reciprocal control of glutamine synthetase and glutaminase B. In contrast ATP is an inhibitor of glutaminase B, while AMP is an activator. Similar regulated enzyme couples exist in the gluconeogenic glycolytic pathway. The same reciprocal controls appear to regulate the activities of fructose 1,6-diphosphatase and phosphofructokinase (Stadtman, 1970). Fructose 1,6-diphosphatase is activated by ATP and inhibited by AMP. Phosphofructokinase is allosterically inhibited by ATP, which is also a substrate, and is activated by AMP. It appears that these potential "futile cycles" provide the organism with enzymatic machinery which can respond to diverse metabolic situations.

Disturbances of ammonia metabolism in mammals

In mammals, several disease states associated with hyperammonemia have been recognized. Hepatic failure (Sherlock, 1968; Walker and Schenker, 1970), disorders of the urea cycle (Shih and Efron, 1972), hyperlysinemia (Ghadimi, 1972), ammonia intoxication (Schenker et al., 1967), diseases of protein intolerance (Malmquist et al., 1971) are all characterized by elevated blood ammonia levels. These pathological processes involve central nervous system dysfunction that may be manifested as seizures, coma, and/or mental retardation. It remains to be established whether or not the changes in the central nervous system function associated with hyperammonemia may in part be directly due to alterations of cerebral glutamate and glutamine metabolism. It is noteworthy that rats, which became comatose after acute ammonia intoxication, showed a reduction of brainstem ATP content by 25% and creatine phosphate content by 70% but showed no alterations in cortical energy stores (Schenker et al., 1967). Other studies have demonstrated frequent alterations of blood and cerebrospinal fluid glutamate and glutamine levels in patients with hyperammonemia, secondary to hepatic failure or a genetic defect (Sherlock, 1968; Shih and Efron, 1972). In addition, methionine sulfoximine, an analog of glutamate, when administered to mice produced a marked decrease in the toxicity of ammonia to the brain even though ammonia concentrations rose significantly (Walker and Schenker, 1970). The results are consistent with the suggestion that some of the toxic effects of ammonia may be due to a localized depletion of cellular energy stores, which are a result of the increased synthesis of glutamine and/or glutamate. Indeed, these events may be similar to those observed in *E. coli* where a 90% reduction in ATP stores was observed upon addition of ammonia to the culture media (Schutt and Holzer, 1972). Recent studies have suggested that the coma associated with hepatic failure may not be due to hyperammonemia but to the synthesis of a false neuro-transmitter, octopamine, because the administration of L-dopa to patients with hepatic coma has resulted in their arousal (Fischer and Baldessarini, 1971).

To date, we are unaware of a deficiency of glutamine synthetase in mammals, but recently a deficiency of glutaminase has been suggested as the cause of a disease, *familial protein intolerance*, associated with hyperammonemia (Malmquist et al., 1971). Further studies are needed to establish the nature of the suspected glutaminase defect in this disease.

In conclusion, the enzymatic control of glutamate and glutamine metabolism in microorganisms is an example of the complex and elegant mechanisms that have evolved to regulate the assimilation and excretion of nitrogenous metabolites. It is hoped that some of this information may be useful in understanding the regulation and functions of nitrogen metabolism in multicellular organisms.

ACKNOWLEDGMENT   With pleasure and appreciation, I thank Dr. Earl Stadtman for his guidance and support throughout these studies.

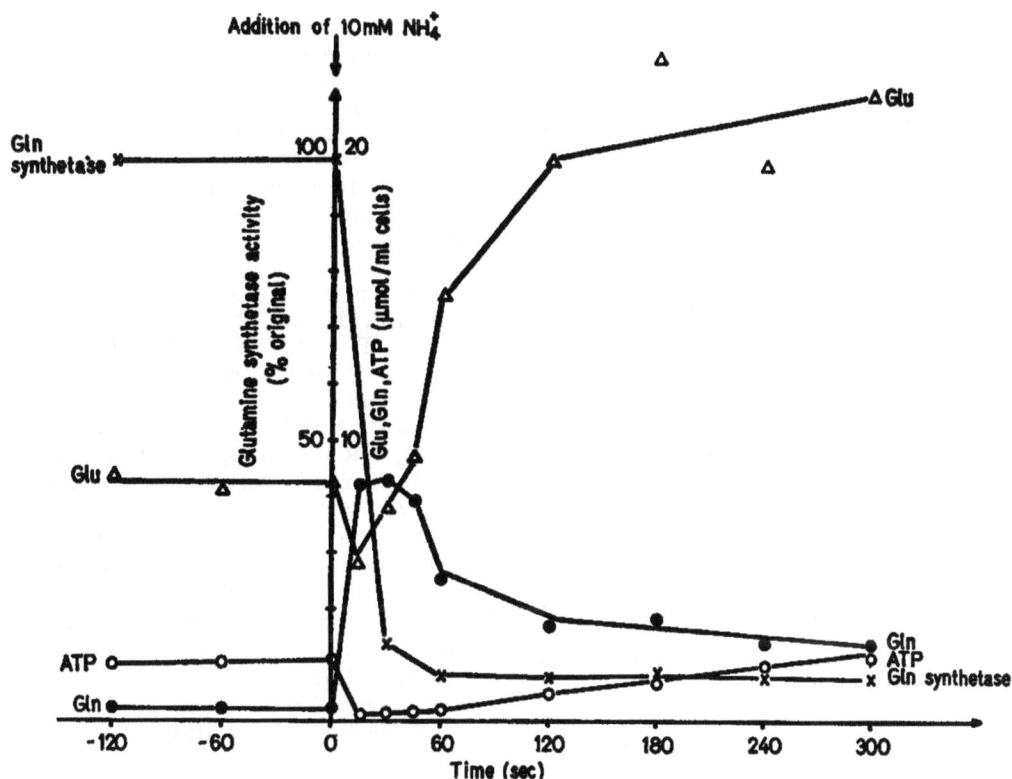

FIGURE 7   Alterations of glutamate, glutamine, ATP content, and glutamine synthetase activity of *E. coli* cells after the addition of 10 mM NH₄⁺ (from Schutt and Holzer, 1972).

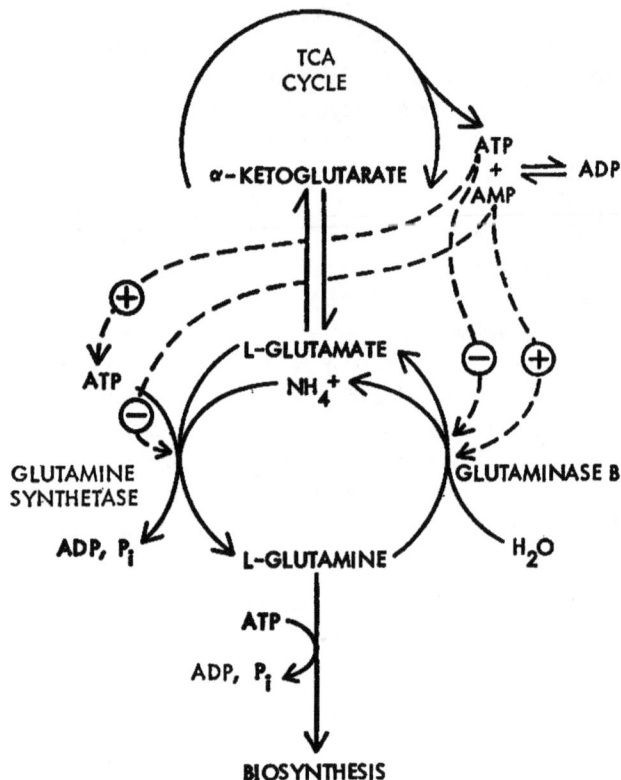

FIGURE 8 Reciprocal control of glutamine synthetase and glutaminase B in *E. coli* by adenine nucleotides.

REFERENCES

BERBERICH, M. A., 1972. A glutamate-dependent phenotype in *E. coli* K12: The result of two mutations. *Biochem. Biophys. Res. Comm.* 47:1498–1503.

BERL, S., and D. D. CLARKE, 1970. Compartmentation of amino acid metabolism. In *Handbook of Neurochemistry*, Vol. 3, Abel Lajtha, ed. New York: Plenum Press, pp. 447–472.

BLOOM, F. E., 1972. Amino acids and polypeptides in neuronal function. *Neurosciences Res. Prog. Bull.* 10:122–251.

BROWN, M. S., A. SEGAL, and E. R. STADTMAN, 1971. Modulation of glutamine synthetase adenylylation and deadenylylation is mediated by metabolic transformation of the P_{II} regulatory protein. *Proc. Nat. Acad. Sci. USA* 68:2949–2953.

CASKEY, C. T., D. ASHTON, and J. WYNGAARDEN, 1964. The enzymology of feedback inhibition of glutamine phosphoribosylpyrophosphate amidotransferase by purine ribonucleotides. *J. Biol. Chem.* 239:2570–2579.

DEUEL, T. F., A. GINSBERG, J. YEH, E. SHELTON, and E. R. STADTMAN, 1970. *Bacillus subtilis* glutamine synthetase. *J. Biol. Chem.* 245:5195–5205.

DEUEL, T., and S. PRUSINER, 1973. *J. Biol. Chem.* (in press).

ELMERICH, C., and J-P. AUBERT, 1971. Synthesis of glutamate by a glutamine: 2-oxo-glutarate amidotransferase (NADP oxidoresductase) in *Bacillus megatherium. Biochem. Biophys. Res. Commun.* 42:371–376.

ELMERICH, C., and J. AUBERT, 1972. Role of glutamine synthetase in the repression of bacterial sporulation. *Biochem. Biophys. Res. Commun.* 46:892–897.

FISCHER, J., and R. BALDESSARINI, 1971. False neurotransmitters and hepatic failure. *Lancet* 2:75–80.

GANCEDO, C., and H. HOLZER, 1968. Enzymatic inactivation of glutamine synthetase in enterobacteriaceae. *Eur. J. Biochem.* 4:190–192.

GHADIMI, H., 1972. The hyperlysinemias. In *Inherited Basis of Metabolic Diseases*, 3rd Ed., J. Stanbury, J. Wyngaarden, and D. Fredrickson, eds. New York: McGraw-Hill, pp. 393–403.

GINSBURG, A., 1969. Conformational changes in glutamine synthetase from *Escherichia coli*. II. Some characteristics of the equilibrium binding of feedback inhibitors to the enzyme. *Biochem.* 8:1726–1740.

HARTMAN, S., 1968. Glutaminase of *Escherichia coli. J. Biol. Chem.* 243:853–863.

HIMWICH, W. A., and H. C. AGRAWAL, 1969. Amino acids. In *Handbook of Neurochemistry*, Vol. 1, Abel Lajtha, ed. New York: Plenum Press, pp. 33–52.

HUBBARD, J., and E. R. STADTMAN, 1967. Regulation of glutamine synthetase. VI. Interactions of inhibitors for *Bacillus licheniformis* glutamine synthetase. *J. Bacteriol.* 94:1016–1024.

JOHNSON, J. L., 1972. Glutamic acid as a synaptic transmitter in the nervous system. A review. *Brain Res.* 37:1–20.

MALMQUIST, J., R. JAGENBERG, and G. LINSTEDT, 1971. Familial protein intolerance. *New Eng. J. Med.* 284:997–1002.

MEERS, J. L., D. W. TEMPEST, and C. M. BROWN, 1970. "Glutamine (amide): 2-oxoglutarate amino transferase oxidoreductase (NADP)," an enzyme involved in the synthesis of glutamate by some bacteria. *J. Gen. Microbiol.* 64:187–194.

MILLER, R. E., and E. R. STADTMAN, 1972. Glutamate synthase from *Escherichia coli*: An iron-sulfide flavoprotein. *J. Biol. Chem.* 247:7407–7419.

MURRELL, W. G., 1969. Chemical composition of spores and spore structures. In *The Bacterial Spore*, G. W. Gould and A. Hurst, eds. New York: Academic Press, pp. 215–273.

PASTAN, I., and R. PERLMAN, 1970. Cyclic adenosine monophosphate in bacteria. *Science* 169:339–344.

PATEMAN, J. A., 1969. Regulation of synthesis of glutamate dehydrogenase and glutamine synthetase in micro-organisms. *Biochem. J.* 115:769–775.

PENNER, P. E., and L. H. COHEN, 1969. Effects of adenosine triphosphate and magnesium ions on the fumarase reaction. *J. Biol. Chem.* 244:1070–1075.

PETERKOFSKY, A., 1972. Personal communication.

PRUSINER, S., R. E. MILLER, and R. C. VALENTINE, 1972. Cyclic AMP control of the enzymes of glutamine metabolism. *Proc. Nat. Acad. Sci. USA* 69:2922–2926.

PRUSINER, S., and E. R. STADTMAN, 1971. On the regulation of glutaminase in *E. coli*: Metabolite control. *Biochem. Biophys. Res. Commun.* 45:1474–1481.

PRUSINER, S., and E. R. STADTMAN, eds., 1973. *The Enzymes of Glutamine Metabolism*. New York: Academic Press, 615 pp.

ROBERTS, E., 1972. Hypothesis: The possible role of GABA in schizophrenia. *Neurosciences Res. Prog. Bull.* 10:468–482.

ROSE, S., 1970. The compartmentation of glutamate and its metabolites in fractions of neuron cell bodies and neuropil: Studied by intraventricular injection of $(U^{14}-C)$ glutamate. *J. Neurochem.* 17:809–816.

SALGANICOFF, L., and E. DE ROBERTIS, 1965. Subcellular distribution of the enzymes of the glutamic acid, glutamine and γ-aminobutyric acid cycles in rat brain. *J. Neurochem.* 12:287–309.

SANWAL, B. D., 1970. Allosteric controls of amphibolic pathways in bacteria. *Bact. Rev.* 34:20–39.

SCHENKER, S., D. MCCANDLESS, E. BROPHY, and M. LEWIS, 1967. Studies on the intracerebral toxicity of ammonia. *J. Clin. Invest.* 46: 838–848.

SCHERAGA, H. W., G. NEMETHY, and I. STEINBERG, 1962. The contribution of hydrophobic bonds to thermal stability of protein conformation. *J. Biol. Chem.* 237: 2506–2508.

SCHUTT, H., and H. HOLZER, 1972. Biological function of the ammonia-induced inactivation of glutamine synthetase in *Escherichia coli. Eur. J. Biochem.* 26: 68–72.

SHERLOCK, S., 1968. *Diseases of the Liver and Biliary System.* Philadelphia, Pa.: F. A. Davis, pp. 79–102.

SHIH, V., and M. EFRON, 1972. Urea cycle disorders. In *Inherited Basis of Metabolic Diseases*, 3rd Ed., J. Stanbury, J. Wyngaarden, and D. Fredrickson, eds. New York: McGraw-Hill, pp. 370–392.

SILVER, S., P. JOHNSEINE, and K. KING, 1970. Manganese active transport in *Escherichia coli. J. Bacteriol.* 104: 1299–1306.

SODERLING, T. R., J. HICKENBOTTOM, E. REIMANN, F. HUNKELER, D. WALSH, and E. KREBS, 1970. Inactivation of glycogen synthetase and activation of phosphorylase kinase by muscle adenosine 3′:5′-monophosphate-dependent protein kinases. *J. Biol. Chem.* 245: 6317–6328.

SOURKES, T. L., 1962. *Biochemistry of Mental Disease.* New York: Harper and Row, pp. 45–60.

STADTMAN, E. R., 1970. Mechanisms of enzyme regulation in metabolism. In *The Enzymes*, Vol. 1, 3rd Ed., P. D. Boyer, ed. New York: Academic Press, pp. 398–460.

STADTMAN, E. R., 1971. The role of multiple molecular forms of glutamine synthetase in the regulation of glutamine metabolism in *Escherichia coli. Harvey Lect.* 65: 97–125.

STADTMAN, E. R., B. SHAPIRO, A. GINSBURG, H. W. KINGDON, and M. DENTON, 1968. Regulation of glutamine synthetase activity in *Escherichia coli. Brookhaven Sympos. Biol.* 21: 378–395.

TRUFFA-BACHI, P., and G. N. COHEN, 1966. La β-aspartokinase sensible à la lysine d'*Escherichia coli* purification et propriétés. *Biochem. Biophys. Acta* 113: 531–541.

VALENTINE, R. C., B. SHAPIRO, and E. R. STADTMAN, 1968. Regulation of glutamine synthetase. XII. Electron microscopy of the enzyme from *Escherichia coli. Biochemistry* 7: 2143–2152.

VAN DEN BERG, C. J., 1970. Glutamate and glutamine. In *Handbook of Neurochemistry*, Vol. 3, Abel Lajtha, ed. New York: Plenum Press, pp. 355–379.

WAELSCH, H., 1951. Glutamic acid and cerebral function. In *Advances in Protein Chemistry*, Vol. 6, M. Anson et al., eds. New York: Academic Press, pp. 299–341.

WALKER, C. O., and S. SCHENKER, 1970. Pathogenesis of hepatic encephalopathy with special reference to the role of ammonia. *Amer. J. Clin. Nutr.* 23: 619–632.

WILCOX, M., 1969. γ-Glutamyl phosphate attached to glutamine-specific t-RNA. *Eur. J. Biochem.* 11: 405–412.

WILLIAMS, A. H., M. H. KYU, J. FENTON, and J. CAVANAGH, 1972. The glutamate and glutamine content of rat brain after portocaval anastomosis. *J. Neurochem.* 19: 1073–1077.

WOOLFOLK, C., and E. R. STADTMAN, 1964. Cumulative feedback inhibition in the multiple end product regulation of glutamine synthetase activity in *Escherichia coli. Biochem. Biophys. Res. Commun.* 17: 313–319.

76 Regulation of the Neurotransmitter Norepinephrine

JULIUS AXELROD

ABSTRACT The catecholamines dopamine, norepinephrine, and epinephrine are in a state of flux, yet they maintain a constant level in nerves and glandular tissues. The level of these biogenic amines is regulated by changes in activity of the biosynthetic enzymes tyrosine hydroxylase, dopamine-β-hydroxylase, and phenylethanolamine-N-methyltransferase. The minute-to-minute regulation of the level of the neurotransmitter norepinephrine is controlled by rapid changes in tyrosine hydroxylase activity caused by feedback inhibition of the enzyme by norepinephrine and dopamine. There is no change in the amount of enzyme protein. Elevation in tyrosine hydroxylase occurs in the cell body, nerve terminals, and adrenal medulla when there is an increase in firing of sympathetic nerves. This results in formation of new enzyme protein by a transsynaptic process. A similar transsynaptic induction by increased nerve firing occurs with the enzyme dopamine-β-hydroxylase in nerves and adrenal medulla. The induction of these enzymes appears to be initiated by acetylcholine and possibly controlled by intracellular concentrations of norepinephrine. The activity of tyrosine hydroxylase and dopamine-β-hydroxylase and especially phenylethanolamine N-methyltransferase in the adrenal medulla is reduced by removal of the pituitary gland and induced by ACTH.

Dopamine-β-hydroxylase is transported from cell body to nerve terminals. When nerves are depolarized, dopamine-β-hydroxylase is released from the nerves, together with the neurotransmitter norepinephrine, by a process of exocytosis. The release of dopamine-β-hydroxylase requires Ca^{++}, microtubules, and microfilaments.

The biogenic amine serotonin undergoes a circadian change in levels in the pineal gland. The level of serotonin is regulated by the neurotransmitter norepinephrine released from sympathetic nerves. Norepinephrine reduces the serotonin levels by stimulating the enzyme that acetylates serotonin via cyclic AMP. Changes in the rate of neuronal release of norepinephrine markedly influence the activity of N-acetyltransferase.

THE ACTIVITY OF the sympathetic nervous system undergoes rapid changes yet maintains a constant level of its neurotransmitter, norepinephrine. This is made possible by a variety of self-regulatory systems involving changes in its biosynthesis, storage, release, and metabolism within the neuron as well as modifications of the pre- and post-

JULIUS AXELROD Laboratory of Clinical Science, National Institute of Mental Health, Bethesda, Maryland

synaptic membrane. The special morphology of the sympathetic neuron also contributes to the maintenance of the neurotransmitter. The sympathetic neuron consists of a cell with a considerable spatial separation from its nerve terminals (Figure 1). The nerve terminals are highly branched and have swellings or varicosities that are in close proximity to the effector cells. Within the varicosity, norepinephrine is stored in a dense core vesicle of about 500 Å (Wolfe et al., 1962). This structural organization is present in both the peripheral and central nervous systems. The cell body of a sympathetic neuron synapses with a preganglionic fiber, usually cholinergic, and the varicosity of the nerve terminals innervates many thousand effector cells *en passant*.

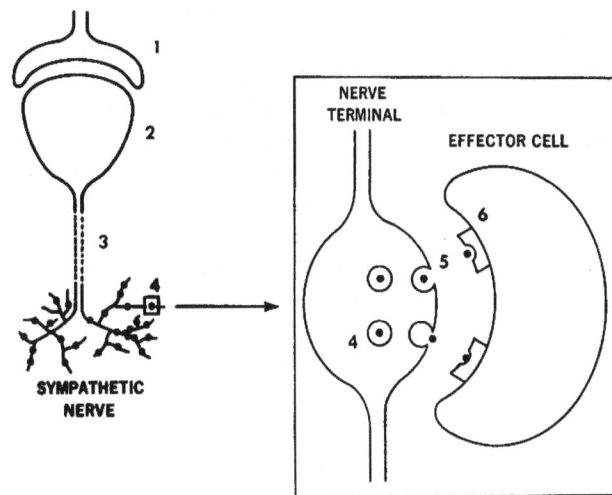

FIGURE 1 Sites at which the neurotransmitter norepinephrine can be regulated (see text for explanation).

The levels of norepinephrine within the sympathetic neuron can be regulated at several sites (Figure 1): Cell body via preganglionic nerves (areas 1, 2); the axon, which transports the biosynthetic enzymes made in the cell body (area 3); the cytoplasm and storage vesicle of nerve terminal (area 4); the neuronal membrane (area 5); and the postsynaptic membrane (area 6).

Biosynthesis of norepinephrine and epinephrine

The enzymes involved in the formation of norepinephrine are synthesized in the cell body of the sympathetic neuron. These enzymes are tyrosine hydroxylase, which converts tyrosine to dopa (Nagatsu et al., 1964), dopa decarboxylase (Holtz et al., 1938), and dopamine-β-hydroxylase, the enzyme that β-hydroxylates dopamine to norepinephrine (Friedman and Kaufman, 1965). Phenylethanolamine-N-methyltransferase, the enzyme that methylates norepinephrine to epinephrine, is present mainly in adrenal medulla of mammals and sympathetic nerves of amphibians (Axelrod, 1962). Tyrosine hydroxylase is a mixed function oxidase requiring tetrahydropteridine and O_2 and Fe^{++}. It is found in the cell body, axon, nerve terminals, as well as the adrenal medulla, and is absent in extraneural tissue. Tyrosine hydroxylase is found in soluble and bound form. A molecular weight of 192,000 has been reported for the soluble enzyme, while the bound enzyme after trypsin digestion has a molecular weight of 50,000 (Wurzburger and Musacchio, 1971). Tyrosine hydroxylase can be inhibited by norepinephrine, which serves as an important controlling mechanism for its synthesis. Inhibition of the enzyme by catecholamines is competitive for its pteridine cofactor in its reduced form and not with its substrate, tyrosine (Ikeda et al., 1966). Dopa decarboxylase is unspecific in that it can decarboxylate a variety of L-aromatic amino acids. It requires pyridoxal phosphate as a cofactor and is tightly bound to the apoenzyme as a Schiff base. Dopa decarboxylase is present both in neuronal and extraneuronal tissues. Using an immunoassay, it was shown that aromatic acid decarboxylase is a single enzyme with a molecular weight of 109,000 (Christenson et al., 1972). Dopamine-β-hydroxylase hydroxylates dopamine on the beta carbon to form norepinephrine. It is a mixed function oxidase containing 2 mole of Cu^{++}, which is reduced by ascorbic acid (Friedman and Kaufman, 1965). The enzyme lacks specificity and can β-hydroxylate a variety of phenylethylamines. The enzyme is highly localized in the sympathetic neuron as well as the adrenal medulla. Within the neuron dopamine-β-hydroxylase is present in the cell body, axon, and nerve terminal. It is highly localized in the norepinephrine storage vesicles of nerves (Potter and Axelrod, 1963a) and chromaffin granules of the adrenal medulla (Kirshner, 1957).

The epinephrine-forming enzyme, phenylethanolamine-N-methyltransferase, is highly localized in the cytoplasm of mammalian adrenal medulla (Axelrod, 1962) and is present in sympathetic nerves of amphibians (Wurtman et al., 1968b). It methylates norepinephrine as well as β-hydroxylated phenylethanolamine derivatives; S-adenosylmethionine is the methyl donor. The enzyme has been purified and its molecular weight has been found to be about 30,000 (Connett and Kirshner, 1970). Phenylethanolamine-N-methyltransferase shows different electrophoretic mobility on starch block, and multiple forms of the enzyme have also been reported (Axelrod and Vesell, 1970). The biosynthesis of catecholamines is shown in Figure 2.

Neural regulation of the catecholamine biosynthetic enzymes

In a study to determine the intraneural localization of tyrosine hydroxylase, 6-hydroxydopamine, a compound that destroys sympathetic nerve terminals (Thoenen and Tranzer, 1968), was administered to rats. There was an almost complete disappearance of this enzyme in the heart in 40 hr suggesting that it was highly localized in sympathetic nerve terminals (Mueller et al., 1969a). When tyrosine hydroxylase was measured in the adrenal gland

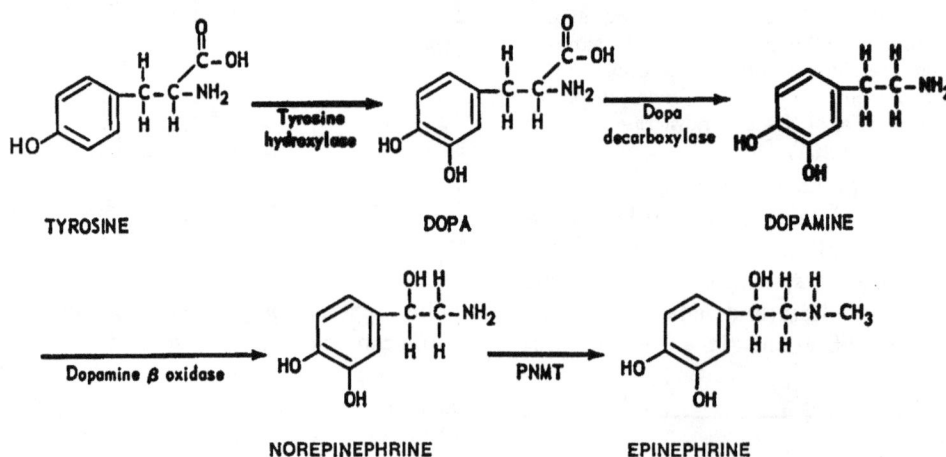

FIGURE 2   Biosynthesis of catecholamines. PNMT is phenylethanolamine N-methyltransferase.

there was a marked increase in this enzyme and a smaller elevation of phenylethanolamine-N-methyltransferase about 1 day after the administration of 6-hydroxydopamine. This was an unexpected finding, and it appeared to be due to the ability of 6-hydroxydopamine to lower blood pressure. This would cause a reflex increase in sympathetic nerve activity, resulting in an increase in enzyme activity in the adrenal gland. To examine this possibility, reserpine and phenoxybenzamine, compounds that lower blood pressure and increase sympathetic nerve activity, were given, and their effects on tyrosine hydroxylase in the adrenal gland examined (Mueller et al., 1969b). Both compounds elevated tyrosine hydroxylase activity, not only in the adrenal gland but also in the superior cervical (Figure 3) and stellate ganglia. The maximal enzyme activity observed in the adrenal gland and the ganglia occurred 3 days after reserpine administration, indicating a slow rise in enzyme activity. Reserpine was also found to increase tyrosine hydroxylase activity in adrenal gland of all mammalian species examined as well as the brainstem of the rabbit. Increased tyrosine hydroxylase activity after reserpine was also observed in the nerve terminal as well as in the cell body. The increase in enzyme activity in the nerve terminal was delayed and lagged behind the rise in the ganglia by 2 days (Thoenen et al., 1970).

The elevation in tyrosine hydroxylase activity after the increase in sympathetic nerve activity was shown physiologically by the increased formation of $[^{14}C]$catechol-amine from $[^{14}C]$tyrosine after the administration of phenoxybenzamine or 6-hydroxydopamine (Dairman and Udenfriend, 1970; Mueller, 1971). The rise in tyrosine hydroxylase activity in the ganglia and adrenal medulla after reserpine administration could be prevented by the administration of cycloheximide or actinomycin D (Mueller et al., 1969c), suggesting that this elevation of enzyme activity is due to induction of new enzyme protein. The Km for both the substrate and the pteridine cofactor with the enzyme obtained from reserpine-treated rats was not different from the untreated rats, although there was a marked elevation in the V_{max} for both substrate and cofactor. These results are consistent with an increase in the number of active sites on the enzyme molecule caused by a drug-induced rise in sympathetic nerve activity. Increased tyrosine hydroxylase activity was found in the adrenal gland after cold (Thoenen et al., 1969a), immobilization (Kvetnansky et al., 1970), and psychosocial stress (Axelrod et al., 1970), in the ganglia after administration of nerve growth factor (Thoenen, 1970), and in brain after cold stress and administration of reserpine (Segal et al., 1971).

To examine whether the induction in tyrosine hydroxylase after reserpine was a transsynaptic event the preganglionic fibers to the superior cervical ganglia (Thoenen et al., 1969a) and the splanchnic nerve to the adrenal gland were cut unilaterally (Thoenen et al., 1969b). When reserpine was administered, there was an elevation

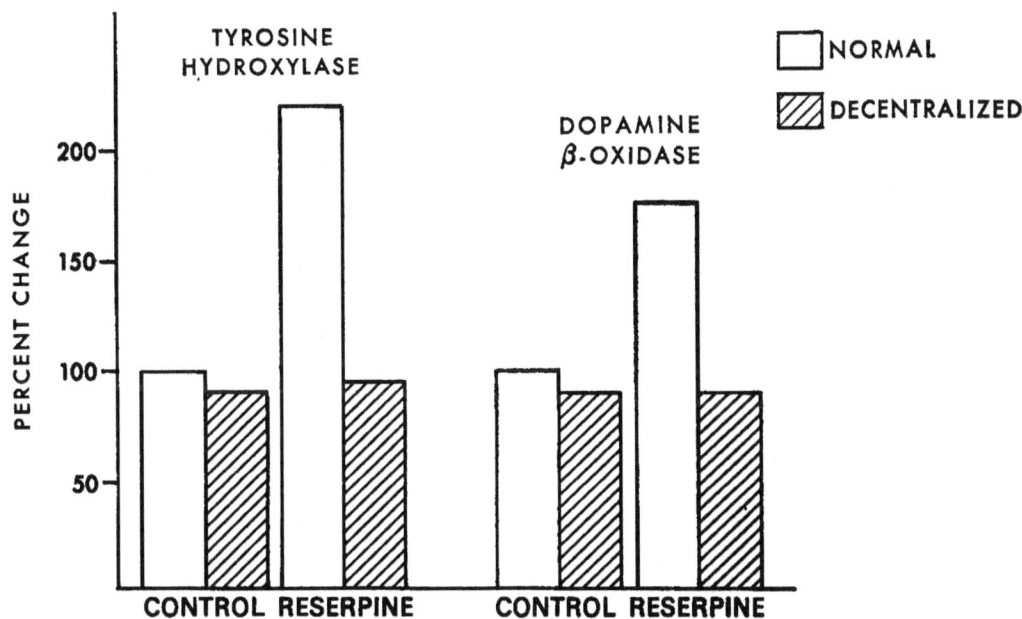

FIGURE 3 Transsynaptic induction of tyrosine hydroxylase and dopamine-β-oxidase(hydroxylase) in sympathetic ganglia. Superior cervical ganglion was decentralized unilaterally by transection of the preganglionic trunk. Two to six days later reserpine (5 mg/kg) was given for 1 day before tyrosine hydroxylase was measured or 3 alternate days before dopamine-β-oxidase(hydroxylase) was measured (from Axelrod, 1971).

of enzyme activity in the innervated side of the ganglia and adrenal gland, but the increase on the denervated side was completely blocked (Figure 3). All of these observations indicate that tyrosine hydroxylase activity is increased in both the sympathetic nerve, cell body, brain, and adrenal medulla by sympathoadrenal hyperactivity. This elevation in tyrosine hydroxylase activity appears to involve a transsynaptic induction of new enzyme molecules.

The presynaptic fibers that regulate tyrosine hydroxylase activity are cholinergic. Interrupting the cholinergic splanchnic nerve blocks the drug-induced rise in tyrosine hydroxylase (Thoenen et al., 1969a, 1969b). Ganglionic blocking agents also inhibit the increase in this enzyme (Mueller et al., 1970b), while acetylcholine causes an elevation of tyrosine hydroxylase activity in the adrenal (Patrick and Kirshner, 1971). In the superior cervical ganglia of the newborn mouse, the development of tyrosine hydroxylase is prevented by cutting the preganglionic cholinergic nerve (Black et al., 1971), suggesting that presynaptic cholinergic terminals regulate the formation of tyrosine hydroxylase in the sympathetic nerve cell body. The selective destruction of sympathetic nerves chemically with 6-hydroxydopamine or immunologically with antiserum to the nerve growth factor prevents the normal development of choline acetyltransferase in presynaptic nerve endings, indicating that postsynaptic adrenergic neurons regulate the biochemical development of presynaptic cholinergic nerves (Black et al., 1971).

Breeding studies are being carried out utilizing reciprocal F_1 and F_2 and dominant recessive backcross generations with respect to the catecholamine biosynthetic enzymes (Ciaranello, unpublished observations). Preliminary results suggest that the genes controlling tyrosine hydroxylase, dopamine-β-hydroxylase and phenylethanolamine-N-methyltransferase are linked. It is possible that the three genes are linked and that a single regulatory locus is responsible for the activity of the three biosynthetic enzymes.

The activity of dopamine-β-hydroxylase is also affected by nerve impulses. The development of a sensitive assay for measuring dopamine-β-hydroxylase made it possible to measure this enzyme in the cell body and nerve terminals and to study changes after drugs that increase sympathetic nerve firing (Molinoff et al., 1971). The administration of reserpine resulted in a marked elevation of dopamine-β-hydroxylase activity in sympathetic ganglia (Figure 3), nerve terminals, and adrenal gland but not in the brain (Molinoff et al., 1970). This increase in enzyme activity in cell bodies is neuronally mediated, because the reserpine could not elevate dopamine-β-hydroxylase activity in a denervated ganglia (Figure 3). Pretreatment of animals with the protein synthesis in-

hibitor, cycloheximide, prevented the rise in enzyme activity in the ganglia. Further evidence that new enzyme protein was induced by nerve impulses comes from the use of an antibody for dopamine-β-hydroxylase. Reserpine caused an increase in the rate of incorporation of [^{3}H]leucine into dopamine-β-hydroxylase measured by immunoabsorption (Hartman et al., 1970).

It appears that nerve depolarization is involved in the induction of dopamine-β-hydroxylase. An increase in the potassium concentration of the media containing rat superior cervical ganglia maintained in organ culture results in a marked increase in dopamine-β-hydroxylase in ganglia (Silberstein et al., 1972). This increase in enzyme activity is inhibited by cycloheximide. Nicotinic antagonists block the induction of dopamine-β-hydroxylase in ganglia after reserpine, suggesting that a cholinergic site is involved (Molinoff et al., 1972). Acetylcholine also increases dopamine-β-hydroxylase activity in the denervated adrenal gland (Patrick and Kirshner, 1971). However, it does not appear that the cholinergic receptor is essential for induction of the enzyme, at least in sympathetic nerves, because elevated potassium concentration can increase enzyme activity in the absence of neuronal influences.

Another biosynthetic enzyme, phenylethanolamine-N-methyltransferase, in the adrenal gland, is regulated by neuronal influences. Increasing splanchnic nerve activity with 6-hydroxydopamine, reserpine, or stress causes a small elevation of phenylethanolamine-N-methyltransferase in the rat adrenal gland (Mueller et al., 1969a) and a large increase in the mouse adrenal (Ciaranello et al., 1972a). This increase can be abolished by transection of the nerve supplying the adrenal gland (Thoenen et al., 1970).

Unlike the other catecholamine biosynthetic enzymes, dopa decarboxylase activity in the superior cervical ganglia or adrenal gland is not induced by drug-mediated increase in preganglionic neural activity (Black et al., 1971). These experiments suggest that tyrosine hydroxylase, dopamine-β-hydroxylase, and phenylethanolamine-N-methyltransferase are linked in a coordinate fashion. Genetic studies also indicate that these enzymes are linked (Ciaranello, unpublished observations).

Several experiments suggest that catecholamines are implicated in the induction of dopamine-β-hydroxylase and tyrosine hydroxylase (Molinoff et al., 1972). Drugs that elevate the level of catecholamines, such as L-dopa, monoamine oxidase inhibitors, and bretylium, inhibit the induction of both tyrosine hydroxylase and dopamine-β-hydroxylase. On the other hand, reduction of catecholamines by α-methyl-paratyrosine or high potassium (Silberstein et al., 1972) results in an induction of dopamine-β-hydroxylase activity.

The nerve terminal may have an important influence on the induction of the catecholamine biosynthetic enzymes in the cell body. Destruction of adrenergic nerve terminals with 6-hydroxydopamine or surgical section of the postganglionic axons causes a long-lasting decrease in dopamine-β-hydroxylase in the superior cervical ganglia (Brimijoin and Molinoff, 1971). 6-Hydroxydopamine administration or a postganglionic section also results in a marked increase in the uptake of [^{3}H]norepinephrine in the sympathetic ganglia (Kopin and Silberstein, 1972). The latter phenomena reflects growth of adrenergic membrane surface. These experiments show that when nerve terminals are destroyed the metabolic machinery of the cell body changes its priorities from the production of enzymes concerned with function to the formation of structural elements required for the restoration of the nerve ending.

Hormonal regulation

In addition to nervous inputs, the corticoids can also influence the biosynthesis of catecholamines. The effects of hormones are principally in the adrenal medulla, a structure that can be considered analogous to the cell body of the sympathetic nervous system. An examination of the effects of hormones on catecholamine formation was prompted by the observation that large amounts of epinephrine are present in the adrenal gland of those species in which the medulla is surrounded by a cortex (Coupland, 1965). This suggested to us that corticoids

present in the cortex might be the compounds that stimulate the methylation of norepinephrine to epinephrine. The experimental design to examine this possibility was to reduce corticoids in adrenal cortex by removal of the pituitary gland in rats and then to measure the activity of phenylethanolamine-N-methyltransferase in the adrenal gland (Wurtman and Axelrod, 1966). When rats were hypophysectomized, there was a gradual and steady decline in the norepinephrine methylating enzyme. After about 7 days, only about 20% of the enzyme activity remained in the adrenal medulla (Figure 4). The administration of either dexamethasone, a potent glucocorticoid, or ACTH restored phenylethanolamine-N-methyltransferase activity to the adrenal gland after several days (Figure 4). Inhibition of protein synthesis blocked the increase in enzyme activity after the administration of dexamethasone. When dexamethasone or ACTH was given repeatedly to normal rats there was no increase in enzyme activity in the adrenal gland. All of these experiments demonstrated that glucocorticoids in the adrenal cortex are necessary to maintain phenylethanolamine-N-methyltransferase activity. There are negligible amounts of phenylethanolamine-N-methyltransferase in sympathetic nerve cell body. When dexamethasone is given to newborn rats, phenylethanolamine-N-methyltransferase appears in the superior cervical ganglia (Ciaranello, Jacobowitz, and Axelrod, unpublished observations). The ability of dexamethasone to induce the methylating enzyme in the ganglia is lost after the rat is 2 weeks old. Dexamethasone also increased

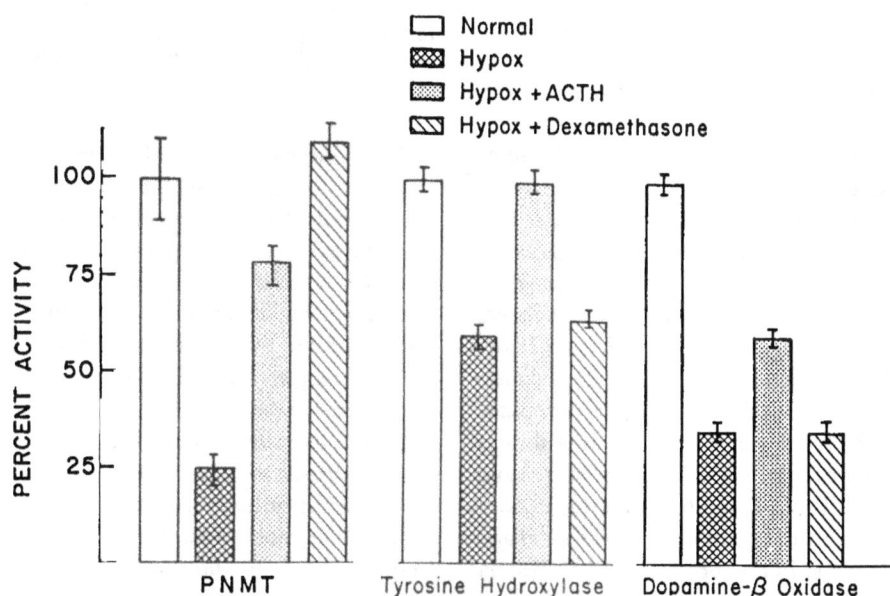

FIGURE 4 Hormonal regulation of catecholamine biosynthetic enzymes in the adrenal. Rats were hypophysectomized for about 1 week and then given dexamethasone or ACTH (from Axelrod, 1973).

the amounts of small, intensely fluorescent (SIF) cells in the superior cervical ganglia. These cells are morphologically related to chromaffin cells. These findings indicate that glucocorticoid hormones may be involved in differentiation of nerve cell to chromaffin type cell .

Removal of the pituitary also affected other catecholamine biosynthetic enzymes in the adrenal medulla. After rat hypophysectomy the activity of tyrosine hydroxylase (Mueller et al., 1970a) and dopamine-β-hydroxylase fell (Weinshilboum and Axelrod, 1970) (Figure 4). Repeated administration of ACTH restored the activity of both enzymes in the adrenal gland (Figure 4). However, dexamethasone failed to elevate tyrosine hydroxylase or dopamine-β-hydroxylase (Figure 4). When mice were subjected to psychosocial stimulation, there was marked elevation of tyrosine hydroxylase and phenylethanolamine-N-methyltransferase in the adrenal gland (Axelrod et al., 1970). When certain mouse strains were exposed to cold stress for 3 to 6 hr, there was a small but significant elevation of phenylethanolamine-N-methyltransferase in the adrenal (Ciaranello et al., 1972a). Implantation of an ACTH-secreting tumor in rats resulted in an elevation of phenylethanolamine-N-methyltransferase, demonstrating that the enzyme can be elevated under conditions of extreme pituitary-adrenocortical activation. Forced immobilization stress also increases tyrosine hydroxylase and dopamine-β-hydroxylase in adrenal to a considerable extent and phenylethanolamine-N-methyltransferase to a smaller degree (Kvetnansky et al., 1970). These stress-induced elevations are mediated by neuronal and hormonal influences.

Regulation of catecholamines at nerve terminals

There is a rapid regulation of the biosynthesis of the adrenergic neurotransmitter in the nerve terminals, which is different from the slower induction of the catecholamine-forming enzymes described above. Stimulation of the splanchnic nerve leads to a release of catecholamines. The sum of the amount of catecholamines released and that remaining in the gland is greater than the amount initially present in the gland (Bydgeman and von Euler, 1958). Studies with the hypogastric nerve (Weiner, 1970) and salivary gland (Sedvall and Kopin, 1967) indicate that the rapid changes in the biosynthesis of norepinephrine are regulated by tyrosine hydroxylase. Stimulation of the sympathetic nerve of the vas deferens in vitro or the salivary gland in vivo (Table I) led to an increased conversion of [^{14}C]tyrosine to [^{14}C]norepinephrine. However, there was no increase in the formation of [^{14}C]dopa to [^{14}C]norepinephrine when the nerves were stimulated, suggesting that tyrosine hydroxylase is the enzyme in-

fluenced by nerve activity. However, there was no increase in the amount of tyrosine hydroxylase in the stimulated salivary gland. In an in vitro study with the vas deferens, it was found that addition of norepinephrine to the bath can partially or completely prevent the increased formation of [^{14}C]norepinephrine from [^{14}C]tyrosine (Weiner, 1970). It has been shown that tyrosine hydroxylase is inhibited by catecholamines such as dopamine and norepinephrine, due to the competition between the catecholamines and the pteridine cofactor (Ikeda et al., 1966). Most of the norepinephrine in the nerve terminals is present in vesicles with little access to tyrosine hydroxylase that appears to be present in the cytoplasm. Thus, there is a small compartment of free catecholamines in the cytoplasm that is critical in the regulation of tyrosine hydroxylase. This small compartment is rapidly depleted during nerve stimulation and thus allows more norepinephrine to be synthesized by increasing the conversion of tyrosine to dopa.

TABLE I

Effect of sympathetic nerve impulses on norepinephrine synthesis and tyrosine hydroxylase activity in the rat salivary gland

	Norepinephrine formed in vivo from		
	[^{14}C]Tyrosine (count/min)	[^{3}H]Dopa (count/min)	In vitro assay of tyrosine hydroxylase*
Decentralized	68	410	3190
Stimulated	358	396	3170

*Tyrosine hydroxylase is expressed as count/min [^{14}C]dopa formed from [^{14}C]tyrosine by an aliquot of homogenate of the salivary glands. (From Sedvall and Kopin, 1967).

Norepinephrine is stored in the nerve terminal in more than one compartment. After the administration of [^{3}H]-norepinephrine, the decrease in its specific activity in tissues was found to be multiphasic (Axelrod et al., 1961), and the specific activity of norepinephrine released by tyramine was dependent on the time the sympathomimetic amine was administered (Potter and Axelrod, 1963b). Kopin et al. (1968) demonstrated that norepinephrine newly synthesized from tyrosine was more rapidly released from the spleen after nerve stimulation. There thus appears to be a relatively small available pool of norepinephrine and a larger reserve store of the catecholamine. The more available pool might be present in the vesicles closest to the synaptic cleft and, because of its location with respect to the neuronal membrane, would be more easily released (Figure 1). The major store of norepinephrine is located at a greater distance from the neuronal membrane and is thus utilized at a slower rate. This pool might serve as a reservoir for the more readily releasable transmitter.

Axonal transport of catecholamine biosynthetic enzymes

The cell body of the sympathetic neuron is separated from the nerve terminals by long distances (Figure 1). The protein-synthesizing apparatus of the neuron is confined to the cell body, while the terminal is involved in nerve function. The enzymes for the biosynthesis of catecholamines made in the cell body must be transported down the axon to the nerve terminal where most of the neurotransmitter is synthesized. Weiss and Hiscoe (1948) demonstrated that the axon is capable of transporting substances from the cell body to the nerve terminal. Axonal transport is a highly specialized process and different constituents are transported in a proximodistal direction at their own characteristic rate, rapidly (1 to 10 mm/hr) or slowly (1 to 3 mm/day) (Ochs, 1972).

Studies on axoplasmic transport are made by ligation of nerves. When adrenergic axons are pinched, there is a rapid accumulation of norepinephrine and dense core vesicles proximal to the constrictions (Dahlström and Häggendal, 1966). When two ligations are made on the same nerve, no accumulation of norepinephrine is observed above the more distal constriction. Colchicine and vinblastine, compounds that cause a disaggregation of microtubules, block the proximodistal transport of dense core vesicles and norepinephrine in noradrenergic neurons (Hökfelt and Dahlström, 1971) implicating microtubules in the rapid axonal transport.

Biochemical and immunological studies indicate that dopamine-β-hydroxylase (Laduron and Belpaire, 1968) and chromogranins, proteins associated with catecholamine binding, also rapidly accumulate proximal to a constriction in peripheral noradrenergic neurons (Geffen et al., 1969). Recently it has been found that dopamine-β-hydroxylase, an enzyme localized in the storage vesicle, and tyrosine hydroxylase, an enzyme not associated with these vesicles, are both transported down the axon of the rat sciatic nerve at an identical rate (1 to 5 mm/hr) (Coyle and Wooten, 1972). Colchicine blocks the transport of both enzymes. These observations suggest that dopamine-β-hydroxylase and tyrosine hydroxylase are transferred from the cell body to the nerve terminal in close association. Local application of colchicine or vinblastine to the superior cervical ganglion of the rat causes a rapid increase in the levels of dopamine-β-hydroxylase in the ganglia and decrease in the salivary gland (Kopin and Silberstein,

1972). When protein synthesis is inhibited the levels of dopamine-β-hydroxylase in the ganglia are rapidly decreased, indicating that the accumulation of the enzyme is due to new synthesis and the decrease after protein synthesis inhibition is the consequence of transport of the enzyme out of the ganglion. Using this approach, the rate of synthesis of dopamine-β-hydroxylase has been calculated to be 5% of the content per hour.

Release of norepinephrine from nerve terminals

The neurotransmitter, norepinephrine, is contained in a membrane-bound vesicle (Wolfe et al., 1962). Thus its discharge from the nerve after depolarization might occur by release into the cytoplasm followed by rapid passage through the neuronal membrane, or by fusion of vesicular membrane with the neuronal membrane and then liberation, or by an opening of the fused membrane and discharge of norepinephrine into the exterior of the terminal together with the soluble contents of the vesicle. This latter process is called *exocytosis*. Evidence that exocytosis occurs comes from studies with adrenal medulla. Stimulation of the adrenal gland with acetylcholine or electrically results in the release of ATP, as well as catecholamines (Douglas and Rubin, 1961). Acetylcholine can also cause the release of the soluble protein of the chromaffin granule, including dopamine-β-hydroxylase (Viveros et al., 1968). The ratio of norepinephrine to dopamine-β-hydroxylase was found to be the same as that present in the chromaffin granule of the adrenal medulla (Viveros et al., 1969). These findings and microscopic evidence indicate that catecholamines are released from the adrenal medulla by a process of exocytosis. When the sympathetic nerve to the spleen is stimulated, dopamine-β-hydroxylase is released together with norepinephrine (Smith et al., 1970). However, the ratio of the amine to dopamine-β-hydroxylase released was 100 times greater than that found in the vesicles isolated from the splenic nerve. Using a very sensitive assay for dopamine-β-hydroxylase, together with the addition of albumin to protect the enzyme, the ratio of dopamine-β-hydroxylase to norepinephrine released after electrical stimulation of the hypogastric nerve of the vas deferens was found to be similar to that in the soluble portion of the contents of the synaptic vesicle (Weinshilboum et al., 1971e). This data indicates that norepinephrine and dopamine-β-hydroxylase are released from the nerve by a process of exocytosis. The absence of Ca^{++} prevents the release of the enzyme and neurotransmitter, while their discharge is enhanced by increasing the concentration of Ca^{++} to twice that used normally (Johnson et al., 1971). The increased release of dopamine-β-hydroxylase with high Ca^{++} concentration is blocked by prostaglandin E$_2$. The α-adrenergic blocking agent, phenoxybenzamine, also increases the release of norepinephrine and dopamine-β-hydroxylase in the stimulated vas deferens, but this drug has no effect on the unstimulated preparation. Prostaglandin also blocks the effects of phenoxybenzamine (Johnson et al., 1971). The enhanced release of dopamine-β-hydroxylase by phenoxybenzamine only when the nerve is stimulated suggests that there is an α-adrenergic receptor on the nerve membrane, and blocking this receptor keeps the nerve membrane in a conformational state that allows larger molecules to be secreted for a longer period of time. Prostaglandins may act by interfering with the actions of Ca^{++} and thus reduce the Ca^{++}-dependent secretion of norepinephrine and dopamine-β-hydroxylase.

Microtubules have been shown to be involved in the discharge of intracellular stored products such as the release of ^{131}I from the thyroid gland (Williams and Wolff, 1970), insulin from the beta cells of the pancreas (Lacy et al., 1968), histamine from mast cells (Gillespie et al., 1968), and catecholamines from the adrenal medulla (Poisner and Bernstein, 1971). These findings suggested that microtubules might play a role in the release of dopamine-β-hydroxylase from sympathetic nerve terminals. Treatment of the vas deferens with colchicine and vinblastine, compounds that disaggregate microtubules, almost completely prevented the release of dopamine-β-hydroxylase and norepinephrine when the nerve is stimulated (Thoa et al., 1972). These compounds, how-

ever, have no effect on the spontaneous release of the enzyme or transmitter. Cytochalasin B, a fungal metabolite that disrupts microfilaments (Carter, 1967), also inhibits the release of norepinephrine and dopamine-β-hydroxylase. These findings suggest that both microtubules and microfilaments are involved in release of norepinephrine and dopamine-β-hydroxylase by exocytosis. Microtubules are presumed to function as a cytoskeleton, and nerve depolarization might affect the microtubules in such a way as to direct the vesicles to the proper site on the neuronal membrane where release occurs (Figure 5). Ca^{++} has also been reported to activate the contractile microfilaments in nonmuscle cells (Wessells et al., 1971). These findings would suggest the presence of a contractile microfilament on the neuronal membrane that is activated by Ca^{++}, which makes an opening in the membrane large enough to allow the soluble contents of the vesicle to be released (Figure 5). Cyclic AMP might also be involved since it has been demonstrated that dibutyryl cyclic AMP and theophylline increase the release of norepinephrine and dopamine-β-hydroxylase after nerve stimulation (Wooten, Thoa, Kopin, and Axelrod, unpublished observation).

Circulating dopamine-β-hydroxylase

The observation that dopamine-β-hydroxylase can be released from the adrenal gland and the nerve terminals prompted an examination of the blood for this enzyme.

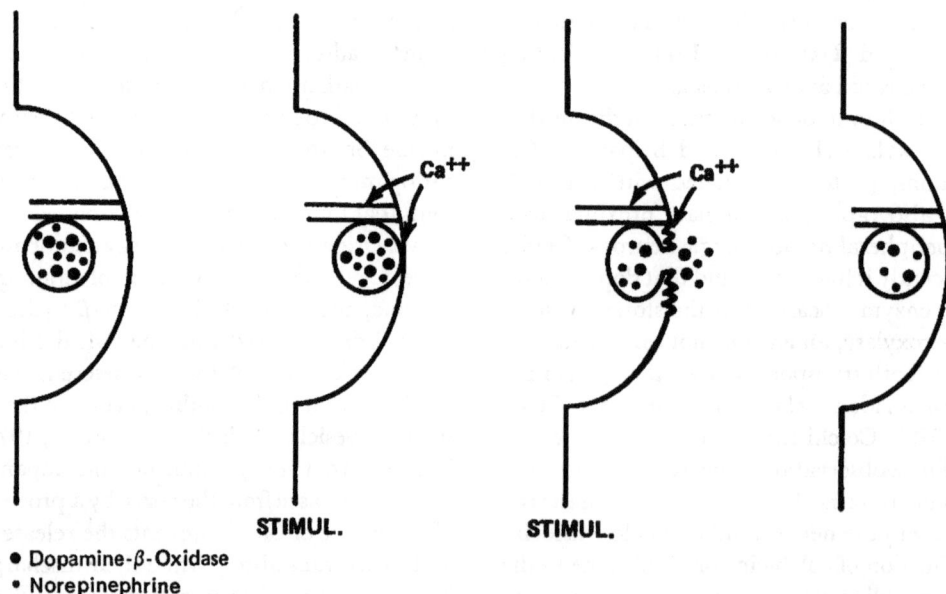

STIMUL.   STIMUL.

● Dopamine-β-Oxidase
• Norepinephrine

FIGURE 5   A possible mechanism for release of norepinephrine and dopamine-β-oxidase (hydroxylase) by exocytosis (see text for explanation). (From Axelrod, 1973).

Dopamine-β-hydroxylase was found to be present in the plasma of man and other mammalian species (Weinshilboum and Axelrod, 1971b; Goldstein et al., 1971).The enzyme in the plasma is similar to purified dopamine β-hydroxylase from the adrenal medulla; both have the same requirements for ascorbic acid, fumarate, and oxygen (Weinshilboum et al., 1971b). They also have similar electrophoretic mobilities and the same Km with respect to substrate.

The plasma dopamine-β-hydroxylase could arise from the sympathetic nerves or the adrenal gland. The administration to rats of 6-hydroxydopamine, a compound that destroys most of the sympathetic nerve terminals but does not affect the adrenal medulla, markedly reduced the level of the plasma dopamine-β-hydroxylase (Weinshilboum and Axelrod, 1971c). On the other hand adrenalectomy did not affect the plasma enzyme levels. The experiments indicate that plasma dopamine-β-hydroxylase comes from sympathetic nerve terminals and that levels of this enzyme in blood suggest a method for measuring activity of these nerves.

In rats subjected to stress, there is an elevation of serum dopamine-β-hydroxylase (Weinshilboum et al., 1971d). When humans were stressed by vigorous exercise or cold pressor test, there was rapid elevation of plasma enzyme. In familial dysautonomia a decrease in plasma dopamine-β-hydroxylase (Weinshilboum and Axelrod, 1971a) is found while subjects with neuroblastoma have an increased enzyme in plasma (Goldstein et al., 1972). Removal of the pituitary gland causes a marked decrease in enzyme activity, which can be prevented by the administration of vasopressin (Lamprecht and Wooten, 1973). This suggests that hypophysectomy, which reduces blood volume, increases sympathetic nerve activity and increases the release of dopamine-β-hydroxylase. Vasopressin increases blood volume and thus results in a reduced sympathetic nerve activity and blood enzyme level.

Regulation of norepinephrine at the neuronal membrane

When norepinephrine is injected into animals it is selectively taken up by sympathetic nerve terminals (Axelrod, 1971; Hertting and Axelrod, 1961). The norepinephrine is then bound in the synaptic vesicle and retained in a physiologically inactive form. This uptake and binding serves as a rapid and effective means of terminating the action of the neurotransmitter. When both monoamine oxidase and catechol-O-methyltransferase, enzymes involved in the metabolism of catecholamines, are inhibited in vivo, the physiological actions

of norepinephrine are only slightly prolonged (Crout, 1961). However, when the uptake of norepinephrine is blocked by drugs (Whitby et al., 1960), or when the sympathetic nerves are destroyed (Hertting et al., 1961b), the response of norepinephrine is considerably increased. These results indicate that uptake of norepinephrine across the neuronal membrane and retention by storage vesicles are a major mechanism for the rapid inactivation of the neurotransmitter (Figure 6).

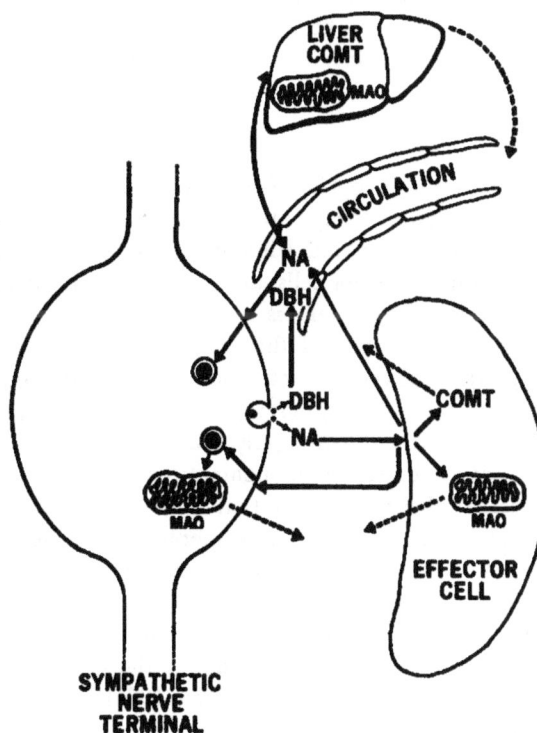

FIGURE 6 Fate of norepinephrine at the sympathetic nerve terminal (see text for explanation). NA is norepinephrine; DBH is dopamine-β-hydroxylase; COMT is catechol-O-methyltransferase; and MAO is monoamine oxidase. (From Axelrod and Weinshilboum, 1972).

The properties of the neuronal uptake mechanism were studied in brain slices (Dengler et al., 1962) and isolated from perfused heart (Iversen, 1963). Uptake of norepinephrine across the neuronal membrane obeys saturation kinetics of the Michaelis-Menten type with high affinity. It also requires sodium ions in the external medium, is temperature dependent, and involves active transport. The uptake process is stereoselective and can be utilized by other phenylethylamine derivatives such as epinephrine, dopamine, tyramine, amphetamine, α-methylnorepinephrine, and meteraminol (Iversen, 1971). High affinity uptake processes similar to norepinephrine's have been demonstrated for other putative neurotransmitters, serotonin, gamma amino butyric acid, glutamate, aspartate, and glycine (Logan and Snyder, 1971).

Norepinephrine can also be taken up by an extraneuronal process (Iversen, 1965; Eisenfeld et al., 1967). This extraneuronal uptake can be blocked by adrenergic blocking agents, normetanephrine (Eisenfeld et al., 1967) and corticosteroids (Iversen, 1971). Compounds such as isoproterenol, which have a low affinity for the intraneuronal uptake and a high affinity for extraneuronal uptake, may be inactivated by the latter process. Extraneuronal uptake may be an important mechanism for removal of the norepinephrine in which the density of the sympathetic innervation is very low or when the synaptic cleft is wide.

Norepinephrine can be inactivated by a variety of mechanisms (Figure 6): Uptake into the neuron, removal by the circulation, enzymatic O-methylation and deamination by liver and kidney, O-methylation and deamination by effector cells, and extraneuronal uptake. Although neuronal uptake is the major mechanism for terminating the action of the sympathetic neurotransmitter, other types of inactivation may predominate, depending on the density of sympathetic innervation, size of the synaptic cleft, blood supply and activity of catechol-O-methyltransferase, and monoamine oxidase.

Several studies have shown that α-adrenergic blocking agents inhibit the uptake of norepinephrine and cause an increased overflow of the neurotransmitter on nerve stimulation (Hertting et al., 1961b; Brown and Gillespie, 1957). It has also been demonstrated that large amounts of endogenous norepinephrine inhibit the discharge of norepinephrine from nerves (Stärke, 1971). These observations suggest another regulatory site on the neuronal membrane. The neuronal membrane appears to have an inhibitory α-adrenergic receptor (Stärke, 1971), which would cause an increased release of the neurotransmitter when the receptor is blocked and a decreased release when a large amount of norepinephrine is present in the synaptic cleft.

Regulation at the postsynaptic effector cell

The sympathetic effector cell could influence the activity of the sympathetic nerve, and conversely the presynaptic cell could influence the activity of the postsynaptic effector cell. When the response of postsynaptic sympathetic effector cells is blocked by phenoxybenzamine, there is a marked increase in tyrosine hydroxylase activity in the adrenal medulla (Thoenen et al., 1969b) and much greater conversion of [^{14}C]tyrosine to [^{14}C]catecholamine (Dairman and Udenfriend, 1970).

Denervation of the sympathetic nerves leads to an increased response of the postsynaptic cell. One explanation for the increased sensitivity is the removal of an important inactivating mechanism; uptake by the neuronal membrane. Another possible mechanism for supersensitivity is an increased responsiveness of the postsynaptic site. It has been shown that in the denervated muscle, the area of binding of α-bungarotoxin, a compound that binds irreversibly to acetylcholine receptors, is increased (Miledi and Potter, 1971).

The pineal cell has been used to study the relationship between the sympathetic nerves and postsynaptic cell. This gland is richly innervated with sympathetic nerves that regulate the synthesis of the hormone melatonin (Wurtman et al., 1968a). Serotonin N-acetyltransferase is an enzyme that N-acetylates serotonin to form the precursor of melatonin (Weissbach et al., 1960). It is present in the postsynaptic pineal cell and is markedly stimulated by norepinephrine and dibutyryl cyclic 3',5'-adenosine monophosphate in organ culture (Klein et al., 1970). In the intact rat, the enzyme activity is also sharply increased after administration of catecholamines (Figure 7) (Deguchi and Axelrod, 1972). The induction of pineal serotonin N-acetyltransferase by catecholamines is prevented by the β-adrenergic blocking agent, propranolol. When the pineal is denervated the catecholamines cause a superinduction (100-fold increase) of serotonin N-acetyltransferase (Figure 7). Although other possibilities have not been excluded, these findings suggest that the increased responsiveness after denervation is due to changes on the postsynaptic β-adrenergic receptor on the pineal cell.

Conclusions

The formation and conservation of the sympathetic neurotransmitter, norepinephrine, is controlled at several sites in the sympathetic neuron. Its synthesis can be rapidly changed by feedback mechanisms on tyrosine hydroxylase in the nerve terminals. Another regulatory site occurs in the cell body and adrenal medulla whereby sympathetic nerve activity changes the rate of formation of various biosynthetic enzymes. Glucocorticoid hormones also influence the synthesis of these enzymes in the adrenal medulla. The biosynthetic enzymes are made in the cell body and transported down the axon to the nerve terminals via proximodistal flow. The transmitter is then synthesized and stored in a vesicle in the nerve terminal. Norepinephrine is released by a process of exocytosis. Once released, the neurotransmitter can be taken up by the nerve terminal and stored and reused again. The presynaptic membrane can affect the activity of the postsynaptic cell by rapidly removing the transmitter by reuptake and influencing the responsiveness of the postsynaptic adrenergic receptor.

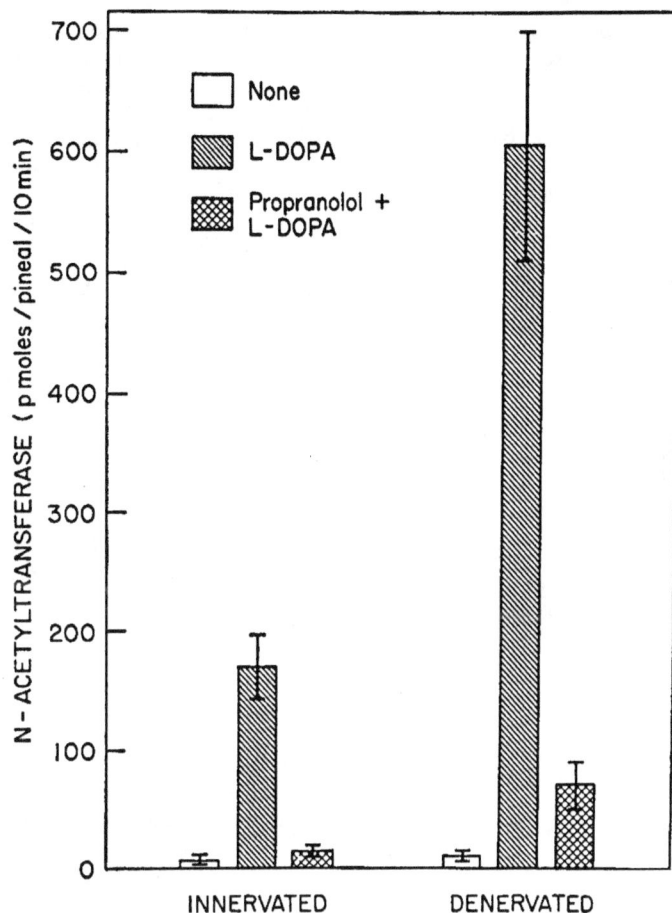

FIGURE 7 Induction and superinduction of serotonin N-acetyltransferase in the rat pineal. Rat pineals were denervated by the bilateral removal of the superior cervical ganglia. Dopa (150 mg/kg) alone or together with propanolol (20 μg/kg) were given at 10 AM and N-acetyltransferase in the pineal was examined 3 hrs later (Deguchi and Axelrod, 1972).

REFERENCES

AXELROD, J., 1962. Purification and properties of phenylethanolamine N-methyltransferase. *J. Biol. Chem.* 237: 1657–1660.

AXELROD, J., 1971. Noradrenaline: Fate and control of its biosynthesis. In *Les Prix Nobel en 1970*, Stockholm: Imprimerieal Royal P. A. Norstedt and Soner, pp. 189–208.

AXELROD, J., 1973. The fate of noradrenaline in the sympathetic neuron. *Harvey Lect.*, Vol. 67, (in press).

AXELROD, J., G. HERTTING, and R. W. PATRICK, 1961. Inhibition of ³H-norepinephrine release by monoamine oxidase inhibitors. *J. Pharmacol. Exp. Ther.* 134:325–328.

AXELROD, J., R. A. MUELLER, J. P. HENRY, and P. M. STEPHENS, 1970. Changes in enzymes involved in the biosynthesis and metabolism of noradrenaline and adrenaline after psychosocial stimulation. *Nature (Lond.)* 225:1059–1060.

AXELROD, J., and E. S. VESELL, 1970. Heterogeneity of N- and O-methyltransferases. *Molec. Pharmacol.* 6:78–84.

AXELROD, J., and R. M. WEINSHILBOUM, 1972. Catecholamines. *New Engl. J. Med.* 287:237–242.

BLACK, I. B., I. HENDRY, and L. L. IVERSEN, 1971. Transsynaptic regulation of growth and development of adrenergic neurons in a mouse sympathetic ganglion. *Brain Res.* 34:229–240.

BRIMIJOIN, S., and P. B. MOLINOFF, 1971. Effects of 6-hydroxydopamine on the activity of tyrosine hydroxylase and dopamine-β-hydroxylase in sympathetic ganglia of the rat. *J. Pharmacol. Exp. Ther.* 178:417–425.

BROWN, G. L., and J. S. GILLESPIE, 1957. The output of sympathetic transmitter from the spleen of the cat. *J. Physiol. (Lond.)* 138:81–102.

BYDGEMAN, S., and U. S. VON EULER, 1958. Resynthesis of catechol hormones in the cat's adrenal medulla. *Acta Phys. Scand.* 44:375–383.

CARTER, S. B., 1967. Effects of cytochalasins on mammalian cells. *Nature (Lond.)* 213:261–264.

CHRISTENSON, J. G., W. DAIRMAN, and S. UDENFRIEND, 1972. On the identity of dopa decarboxylase and 5-hydroxytryptophan decarboxylase. *Proc. Natl. Acad. Sci. USA* 69:343–347.

CIARANELLO, R. D., J. N. DORNBUSCH, and J. D. BARCHAS, 1972a. Rapid increase of phenylethanolamine-N-methyltransferase by environmental stress in an inbred mouse strain. *Science* 175:789–790.

CIARANELLO, R. D., J. N. DORNBUSCH, and J. D. BARCHAS,

1972b. Regulation of adrenal phenylethanolamine N-methyltransferase in three inbred linked mouse strains. *Molec. Pharmacol.* 8:511–519.

CONNETT, R. T., and N. KIRSHNER, 1970. Purification and properties of bovine phenylethanolamine N-methyltransferase. *J. Biol. Chem.* 245:329–334.

COUPLAND, R. E., 1965. *The Natural History of the Chromaffin Cell.* London: Longmans.

COYLE. J. T., and G. F. WOOTEN, 1972. Rapid axonal transport of tyrosine hydroxylase and dopamine-β-hydroxylase. *Brain Res.*, 44:701–704.

CROUT, J. R., 1961. Effect of inhibiting both catechol-O-methyltransferase and monoamine oxidase on the cardiovascular responses to noradrenaline. *Proc. Soc. Exp. Biol. Med.* 108:482–484.

DAHLSTRÖM, A., and J. HÄGGENDAL, 1966. Studies on the transport and life span of amine storage granules in a peripheral adrenergic neuron system. *Acta Physiol. Scand.* 67:278–288.

DAIRMAN, W., and S. UDENFRIEND, 1970. Increased conversion of tyrosine to catecholamines in the intact rat following elevation of tissue tyrosine hydroxylase levels by administered phenoxybenzamine. *Molec. Pharmacol.* 6:350–356.

DEGUCHI, T., and J. AXELROD, 1972. Induction and superinduction of serotonin N-acetyltransferase by adrenergic drugs and denervation in the rat pineal organ. *Proc. Nat. Acad. Sci. USA* 69:2208–2211.

DENGLER, H. J., I. A. MICHAELSON, H. E. SPIEGAL, and E. TITUS, 1962. Uptake of labeled norepinephrine by isolated brain and other tissues of the cat. *Int. J. Neuropharmacol.* 1:23–38.

DOUGLAS, W. W., and R. P. RUBIN, 1961. The role of calcium in the secretory response of the adrenal medulla to acetylcholine. *J. Physiol. (Lond.)* 159:40–57.

EISENFELD, A. J., L. LANDSBERG, and J. AXELROD, 1967. Effect of drugs on the accumulation and metabolism of extraneuronal norepinephrine in the rat heart. *J. Pharmacol. Exp. Ther.* 158:378–385.

FRIEDMAN, S., and S. KAUFMAN, 1965. 3,4-Dihydroxyphenylethylamine β-hydroxylase: Physical properties, copper content and role of copper in the catalytic activity. *J. Biol. Chem.* 240:4763–4773.

GEFFEN, L. B., B. G. LIVETT, and R. A. RUSH, 1969. Immunohistochemical localization of protein components of catecholamine storage vesicles. *J. Physiol. (Lond.)* 204:593–605.

GILLESPIE, E., R. J. LEVINE, and S. E. MALAWISTA, 1968. Histamine release from rat peritoneal mast cells: Inhibition by colchicine and potentiation by deuterium oxide. *J. Pharmacol. Exp. Ther.* 164:158–165.

GOLDSTEIN, M., L. S. FREEDMAN, A. C. BOHUON, and F. GUERINOT, 1972. Serum dopamine-β-hydroxylase in patients with neuroblastoma. *New Engl. J. Med.* 286:1123–1125.

GOLDSTEIN, M., L. S. FREEDMAN, and M. BONNAY, 1971. An assay for dopamine-β-hydroxylase activity in tissues and serum. *Experientia* 27:632–633.

HARTMAN, B. K., P. B. MOLINOFF, and S. UDENFRIEND, 1970. Increased rate of synthesis of dopamine-β-hydroxylase in adrenals of reserpinized rats. *The Pharmacologist* 12:470.

HERTTING, G., and J. AXELROD, 1961. The fate of tritiated noradrenaline at the sympathetic nerve ending. *Nature (Lond.)* 192:172–173.

HERTTING, G., J. AXELROD, I. J. KOPIN, and L. G. WHITBY, 1961a. Lack of uptake of catecholamines after chronic denervation of sympathetic nerves. *Nature (Lond.)* 189:66.

HERTTING, G., J. AXELROD, and L. G. WHITBY, 1961b. Effect of drugs on the uptake and metabolism of ^{3}H-norepinephrine. *J. Pharmacol. Exp. Ther.* 134:146–153.

HÖKFELT, T., and A. DAHLSTRÖM, 1971. Effects of two mitosis inhibitors (colchicine and vinblastine) on the distribution and axonal transport of noradrenaline storage particles. *Z. Zellforsch.* 119:460–482.

HOLTZ, P., R. HEISE, and K. LUDTKE, 1938. Quantitativer abbau von L-Dioxyphenylalanin (Dopa) durch Niere. *Arch. Exp. Path. Pharmak.* 191:87–118.

IKEDA, M., L. A. FAHIEN, and S. UDENFRIEND, 1966. A kinetic study of bovine adrenal tyrosine hydroxylase. *J. Biol. Chem.* 241:4452–4456.

IVERSEN, L. L., 1971. Role of transmitter uptake mechanisms in synaptic neurotransmission. *Brit. J. Pharmacol.* 41:571–591.

IVERSEN, L. L., 1965. The uptake of catecholamines at high perfusion concentrations in the rat isolated heart: A novel catecholamine uptake process. *Brit. J. Pharmacol.* 25:18–33.

IVERSEN, L. L., 1963. The uptake of noradrenaline by the isolated perfused rat heart. *Brit. J. Pharmacol.* 21:523–537.

JOHNSON, D. G., N. B. THOA, R. M. WEINSHILBOUM, J. AXELROD, and I. J. KOPIN, 1971. Enhanced release of dopamine-β-hydroxylase from sympathetic nerves by calcium and phenoxybenzamine and its reversal by prostaglandins. *Proc. Natl. Acad. Sci. USA* 68:2227–2230.

KIRSHNER, N., 1957. Pathway of noradrenaline formation from dopa. *J. Biol. Chem.* 226:821–825.

KLEIN, D. C., G. R. BERG, and J. WELLER, 1970. Melatonin synthesis: Adenosine 3',5'-monophosphate and norepinephrine stimulate N-acetyltransferase. *Science* 168:979–980.

KOPIN, I. J., G. R. BREESE, K. R. KRAUSS, and V. K. WEISE, 1968. Selective release of newly synthesized norepinephrine from the cat spleen during sympathetic nerve stimulation. *J. Pharmacol. Exp. Ther.* 161:271–278.

KOPIN, I. J., and S. D. SILBERSTEIN, 1972. Axons of sympathetic neurons: Transport of enzymes in vivo and properties of axonal sprouts in vitro. *Pharmacol. Rev.* 24:245–254.

KVETNANSKY, R., V. K. WEISE, and I. J. KOPIN, 1970. Elevation of adrenal tyrosine hydroxylase and phenylethanolamine N-methyltransferase by repeated immobilization of rats. *Endocrinology* 87:744–749.

LACY, P. E., S. L. HOWELL, D. A. YOUNG, and C. J. FINK, 1968. New hypothesis of insulin secretion. *Nature (Lond.)* 219:1177–1179.

LADURON, P., and F. BELPAIRE, 1968. Transport of noradrenaline and dopamine-β-hydroxylase in sympathetic nerves. *Life Sci.* 7:1–9.

LAMPRECHT, F., and G. F. WOOTEN, 1973. Effect of hypophysectomy on serum dopamine-β-hydroxylase activity in rat. *Endocrinology* 92: (in press).

LOGAN, W. J., and S. H. SNYDER, 1971. Unique high affinity uptake systems for glycine, glutamic and aspartic acids in central nervous tissue of the rat. *Nature (Lond.)* 234:297–298.

MILEDI, R., and L. T. POTTER, 1971. Acetylcholine receptors in muscle fibers. *Nature (Lond.)* 233:599–603.

MOLINOFF, P. B., S. BRIMIJOIN, and J. AXELROD, 1972. Induction of dopamine-β-hydroxylase and tyrosine hydroxylase in rat hearts and sympathetic ganglia. *J. Pharmacol. Exp. Ther.* 182:116–130.

MOLINOFF, P. B., W. S. BRIMIJOIN, R. M. WEINSHILBOUM, and J. AXELROD, 1970. Neurally mediated increase in dopamine-β-hydroxylase activity. *Proc. Nat. Acad. Sci. USA* 66:453–458.

MOLINOFF, P. B., R. M. WEINSHILBOUM, and J. AXELROD, 1971. A sensitive enzymatic assay for dopamine-β-hydroxylase. *J. Pharmacol. Exp. Ther.* 178:425–531.

MUELLER, R. A., 1971. Effect of 6-hydroxydopamine on the synthesis and turnover of catecholamines and proteins in the adrenal. In *6-Hydroxydopamine and Catecholamines*, T. Malmfors and H. Thoenen, eds. Amsterdam: Elsevier, pp. 291–301.

MUELLER, R. A., H. THOENEN, and J. AXELROD, 1969a. Adrenal tyrosine hydroxylase: Compensatory increase in activity after chemical sympathectomy. *Science* 163:468–469.

MUELLER, R. A., H. THOENEN, and J. AXELROD, 1969b. Increase in tyrosine hydroxylase activity after reserpine administration. *J. Pharmacol. Exp. Ther.* 169:74–79.

MUELLER, R. A., H. THOENEN, and J. AXELROD, 1969c. Inhibition of trans-synaptically increased tyrosine hydroxylase activity by cycloheximide and actinomycin D. *Molec. Pharmacol.* 5:463–469.

MUELLER, R. A., H. THOENEN, and J. AXELROD, 1970a. Effect of pituitary and ACTH on the maintenance of basal tyrosine hydroxylase activity in the rat adrenal gland. *Endocrinology* 86:751–755.

MUELLER, R. A., H. THOENEN, and J. AXELROD, 1970b. Inhibition of neuronally induced tyrosine hydroxylase by nicotinic receptor blockade. *Eur. J. Pharmacol.* 10:51–56.

NAGATSU, T., M. LEVITT, and S. UDENFRIEND, 1964. Tyrosine hydroxylase: The initial step in norepinephrine biosynthesis. *J. Biol. Chem.* 239:2910–2917.

OCHS, S., 1972. Fast transport of materials in mammalian nerve fibers. *Science* 176:252–259.

PATRICK, R. L., and N. KIRSHNER, 1971. Effect of stimulation on the levels of tyrosine hydroxylase, dopamine-β-hydroxylase and catecholamines in intact and denervated rat adrenal glands. *Molec. Pharmacol.* 7:87–96.

POISNER, A. M., and J. BERNSTEIN, 1971. A possible role of microtubules in catecholamine release from the adrenal medulla: Effect of colchicine, vinca alkaloids and deuterium oxide. *J. Pharmacol. Exp. Ther.* 177:102–108.

POTTER, L. T., and J. AXELROD, 1963a. Properties of noradrenaline storage particles of the rat heart. *J. Pharmacol. Exp. Ther.* 142:291–305.

POTTER, L. T., and J. AXELROD, 1963b. Studies on the storage of norepinephrine and the effect of drugs. *J. Pharmacol. Exp. Ther.* 140:199–206.

SEDVALL, G. C., and I. J. KOPIN, 1967. Acceleration of norepinephrine synthesis in the rat submaxillary gland in vivo during sympathetic nerve stimulation. *Life Sci.* 6:45–51.

SEGAL, D. S., J. L. SULLIVAN, R. T. KUCZENSKI, and A. J. MANDELL, 1971. Effects of long-term reserpine treatment on brain tyrosine hydroxylase and behavioral activity. *Science* 173:847–849.

SILBERSTEIN, S. D., S. BRIMIJOIN, P. B. MOLINOFF, and L. LEMBERGER, 1972. Induction of dopamine-β-hydroxylase in rat superior cervical ganglia in organ culture. *J. Neurochem.* 19:919–921.

SMITH, A. D., W. P. DEPOTTER, E. J. MOERMAN, and A. F. DE SCHAEPDRYVER, 1970. Release of dopamine-β-hydroxylase and chromogranin A upon stimulation of the splenic nerve. *Tissue and Cell* 2:547–568.

STÄRKE, K., 1971. Influence of α-receptor stimulants on noradrenaline release. *Naturwissenschaften* 58:420.

THOA, N. B., G. F. WOOTEN, J. AXELROD, and I. J. KOPIN, 1972. Inhibition of release of dopamine-β-hydroxylase and norepinephrine from sympathetic nerves by colchicine, vin-blastine and cytochalasin B. *Proc. Nat. Acad. Sci. USA* 69:520–522.

THOENEN, H., 1970. Induction of tyrosine hydroxylase in peripheral and central adrenergic neurons by cold exposure of rats. *Nature (Lond.)* 228:861–862.

THOENEN, H., R. A. MUELLER, and J. AXELROD, 1969a. Increased tyrosine hydroxylase activity after drug-induced alteration of sympathetic transmission. *Nature (Lond.)* 221:1264.

THOENEN, H., R. A. MUELLER, and J. AXELROD, 1969b. Trans-synaptic induction of adrenal tyrosine hydroxylase. *J. Pharmacol. Exp. Ther.* 169:249–254.

THOENEN, H., R. A. MUELLER, and J. AXELROD, 1970. Neuronally dependent induction of adrenal phenylethanolamine N-methyltransferase by 6-hydroxydopamine. *Biochem. Pharmacol.* 19:669–673.

THOENEN, H., and J. P. TRANZER, 1968. Chemical sympathectomy by selective destruction of adrenergic nerve endings with 6-hydroxydopamine. *Naunyn-Schmiedeberg Arch. Pharm. Exp. Path.* 281:271–288.

VIVEROS, O. H., L. ARQUEROS, R. J. CONNETT, and N. KIRSHNER, 1969. Mechanism of secretion from the adrenal medulla IV. Fate of the storage vesicles following insulin and reserpine administration. *Molec. Pharmacol.* 5:69–82.

VIVEROS, O. H., L. ARQUEROS, and N. KIRSHNER, 1968. Release of catecholamines and dopamine-β-hydroxylase from the adrenal medulla. *Life Sci.* 7:609–618.

WEINER, N., 1970. Regulation of norepinephrine biosynthesis. *Ann. Rev. Pharmacol.* 10:273–290.

WEINSHILBOUM, R., and J. AXELROD, 1970. Dopamine-β-hydroxylase activity in the rat after hypophysectomy. *Endocrinology* 87:894–899.

WEINSHILBOUM, R., and J. AXELROD, 1971a. Reduced plasma dopamine-β-hydroxylase in familial dysautonomia. *New Engl. J. Med.* 285:938–942.

WEINSHILBOUM, R., and J. AXELROD, 1971b. Serum dopamine-β-hydroxylase activity. *Circ. Res.* 28:307–315.

WEINSHILBOUM, R., and J. AXELROD, 1971c. Serum dopamine-β-hydroxylase: Decrease after chemical sympathectomy. *Science* 173:931–934.

WEINSHILBOUM, R., R. KVETNANSKY, J. AXELROD, and I. J KOPIN, 1971d. Elevation of serum dopamine-β-hydroxylase activity with forced immobilization. *Nature New Biology* 230:287–288.

WEINSHILBOUM, R., N. B. THOA, D. G. JOHNSON, I. J. KOPIN, and J. AXELROD, 1971e. Proportional release of norepinephrine and dopamine-β-hydroxylase from the sympathetic nerves. *Science* 174:1349–1351.

WEISS, P., and H. HISCOE, 1948. Experiments on the mechanism of nerve growth. *J. Exp. Zool.* 107:315–396.

WEISSBACH, H., B. G. REDFIELD, and J. AXELROD, 1960. Biosynthesis of melatonin: Enzymic conversion of serotonin to N-acetylserotonin. *Biochim. Biophys. Acta* 43:352–353.

WESSELLS, N. K., B. S. SPOONER, J. F. ASH, M. BRADLEY, M. A. LADUENA, E. L. TAYLOR, J. T. WRENN, and K. M. YAMADA, 1971. Microfilaments in cellular and developmental processes. *Science* 171:135–143.

WHITBY, L. G., G. HERTTING, and J. AXELROD, 1960. Effect of cocaine on the disposition of noradrenaline labeled with tritium. *Nature (Lond.)* 187:604–605.

WILLIAMS, J. A., and J. WOLFF, 1970. Possible role of microtubules in thyroid secretion. *Proc. Nat. Acad. Sci. USA* 67:1901–1908.

WOLFE, D. E., L. T. POTTER, K. C. RICHARDSON, and J. AXELROD, 1962. Localizing tritiated norepinephrine in sympathetic axons by electron microscopic autoradiography. *Science* 138:440–442.

WURTMAN, R. J., and J. AXELROD, 1966. Control of enzymatic synthesis of adrenaline in the adrenal medulla by adrenal cortical steroids. *J. Biol. Chem.* 241:2301–2305.

WURTMAN, R. J., J. AXELROD, and D. E. KELLEY, 1968a. *The Pineal.* New York: Academic Press.

WURTMAN, R. J., J. AXELROD, E. S. VESELL, and G. T. ROSS, 1968b. Species differences in inducibility of phenylethanolamine N-methyltransferase. *Endocrinology* 82:584–590.

WURZBURGER, R. J., and J. M. MUSACCHIO, 1971. Subcellular distribution and aggregation of bovine adrenal tyrosine hydroxylase. *J. Pharmacol. Exp. Ther.* 177:155–157.

77 Development of the Central Catecholaminergic Neurons

JOSEPH T. COYLE, JR.

ABSTRACT The biochemical aspects of the development of the central catecholaminergic neurons have been examined in the rat brain. The high-affinity uptake mechanism for norepinephrine, which is localized at the terminal of the noradrenergic neuron, was used as a specific marker for the neuronal membrane. The uptake mechanism was first demonstrable in the brain at 18 days gestation; during subsequent maturation, its specific activity increased almost fivefold. The increase in uptake of ^{3}H-norepinephrine correlated with an increased localization of the ^{3}H-norepinephrine in the synaptosomal fractions on continuous sucrose gradients.

Tyrosine hydroxylase, dopa decarboxylase, and dopamine-β-hydroxylase, the enzymes in the biosynthetic pathway for norepinephrine, were present in the brain at 15 days gestation. During subsequent development, there was a coordinate increase in the activity of these enzymes in the whole brain. With maturation, there was a translocation of enzyme activity from the regions that contain the cell bodies of the catecholaminergic neurons to those regions that contain only terminals of these neurons. Concurrently, there was an absolute increase in the activity of these enzymes in the synaptosomal fractions. The time at which cell division of the central catecholaminergic neurons ceases has been investigated by means of ^{3}H-thymidine autoradiography; thus, changes in enzyme activity could be more accurately expressed in terms of this specific population of neurons.

Histofluorescent studies done by Loizou and Maeda indicate that, just prior to birth, catecholamine fluorescence is limited to the cell bodies of the catecholaminergic neurons in the brainstem, and that with maturation there is a marked outgrowth of fluorescent fibers innervating the distal regions of the brain. The temporal-spatial changes in the activity of the uptake mechanism, as well as the specific enzymes for the catecholaminergic neurons, offer excellent correlates with these histochemical observations.

Introduction

THE DEVELOPING nervous system provides a scenario in which the complex relationships among neurons take form. This process involves cell multiplication, cell migration, outgrowth of neuronal processes, and synaptogenesis. In abstract terms, the development of the brain is a vectorial process characterized by changes in time and space as well as magnitude (Jacobson, 1970). Research on the development of the mammalian brain has been oriented primarily toward structural analysis, and the correlation between morphologic and biochemical differentiation has remained an elusive goal.

Because of the following factors, the central catecholaminergic neurons of the rat brain may be uniquely susceptible to the elucidation of the complex relationship between morphogenesis and biochemical differentiation. First, a specific histofluorescent technique has been devised whereby the catecholaminergic neurons can be identified in sections of brain tissue (Falck and Hillarp, 1959). The method is based on the fact that the catecholamines within the neurons interact with paraformaldehyde vapor to form a fluorophor that can be visualized by fluorescent microscopy. With this method, the aminergic neuronal pathways have been mapped out in the adult rat brain (Fuxe et al., 1970; Ungerstedt, 1971). Second, the cell bodies of the catecholaminergic neurons are limited to the brainstem although their axons and terminals ramify to innervate other regions of the brain. Thus, properties related to the perikarya can be anatomically distinguished from those related to the axons and terminals. Finally, the enzymatic processes involved in the synthesis and metabolism of catecholamines as well as the pharmacologic properties of these neurons have been well characterized in the adult rat brain (Molinoff and Axelrod, 1971).

Morphogenesis

Catecholamine-induced fluorescence can be observed in the cells that form the noradrenergic nucleus, the locus coeruleus, at 14 days of gestation; over the next 4 days, the neurons migrate caudally to their ultimate position in the pons (Maeda and Dresse, 1969). Fluorescence of the cell bodies of the dopaminergic neurons of the midbrain is apparent at 18 days of gestation, whereas the dopaminergic cell bodies in the hypothalmus first exhibit catecholamine-fluorescence early in the postnatal period (Loizou, 1971; Smith and Simpson, 1970). Thus, there is an apparent caudal-to-rostral sequence of appearance of

JOSEPH T. COYLE, JR. Laboratory of Clinical Science, National Institute of Mental Health, Bethesda, Maryland catecholamine-induced fluorescence in the cell bodies that give rise to the various aminergic neuronal pathways of the brain.

Loizou (1972) has investigated the postnatal development of the aminergic neurons of the rat brain with the histofluorescent technique (Table I). At birth, there is a striking scarcity of noradrenergic terminals, whereas scattered islands of dopaminergic terminals are already present in the caudate nucleus. During the first week after birth, there is a marked increase in the size and fluorescent intensity of the catecholaminergic cell bodies; certain groups of neurons exhibit even more intense fluorescence than observed in the adult. Between the second and third week after birth, the noradrenergic terminals attain an adult pattern of density and intensity of fluorescence in the spinal cord and medulla-pons, whereas the adult pattern is established in the more rostral regions only by the fourth to fifth postnatal week. Although the diffusely intense fluorescence of the dopaminergic terminals in the striatum is maximal by 4 weeks after birth, during subsequent maturation there is a shift in the fluorescent spectrum suggesting further increases in the dopamine concentration. This impression of a more rapid maturation of the noradrenergic neurons as compared to the dopaminergic neurons is substantiated by the fact that norepinephrine attains adult concentration prior to dopamine (Agrawal et al., 1968; Breese and Traylor, 1972; Loizou and Salt, 1970). Thus, two phases in the morphogenesis of the catecholaminergic neurons can be distinguished: A fetal and early postnatal period when the cell bodies acquire catecholamine fluorescence and then a period, primarily postnatal, when there is a centrifugal outgrowth of axons and terminals from the cell bodies.

Time of origin of the catecholaminergic neurons

Maturation of the brain involves multiplication and differentiation of heterogeneous populations of cells. In order to quantify accurately the development of the central catecholaminergic neurons on a "per neuron" basis, it is essential to know when the brain has attained its full complement of these neurons. In other words, at what point in development do the central catecholaminergic neurons cease dividing and start differentiating? Autoradiographic studies of the incorporation of ^{3}H-thymidine have proved to be an accurate method for dating the time of origin of neurons since the radio-labeled thymidine is only incorporated into the DNA of dividing cells (Altman, 1966).

By combining the histofluorescent technique with ^{3}H-thymidine autoradiography, it has been possible to demonstrate when the central catecholaminergic neurons undergo cell division (Nicholson, Coyle, Das, and Bloom, in preparation). The noradrenergic neurons in the locus coeruleus and the dopaminergic neurons in the substantia nigra exhibit a brief period of cell division between 12 and 14 days of gestation and do not divide subsequently. Thus, the two major catecholaminergic nuclei of the brain attain their full complement of neurons a week before birth, and a more appropriate representation of their developmental changes after this date would be on the basis of whole brain activity.

Neuronal membrane uptake process

The catecholaminergic neurons possess on their neuronal membrane a high-affinity uptake mechanism for catecholamines (Axelrod, 1965). This transport mechanism, which is an active process linked to Na$^+$-K$^+$ ATPase, plays a primary role in the inactivation of catecholamines released at the synapse (Tissari et al., 1969; White and Keen, 1970). The uptake mechanism, being highly concentrated in the terminal boutons, can be demonstrated in sheared-off nerve terminals or synaptosomes (Davis et al., 1967). The central dopaminergic and noradrenergic neurons have uptake mechanisms specific for their re-

TABLE I

Density of catecholaminergic terminals in regions of brain during development

	Birth	1 Week	2 Weeks	3 Weeks	Adult
Medulla-pons	0 – few	1 – 2	2 – 3	4	4
Cerebellum	0	1 – 3	1 – 3	few	few
Mesencephalon	0	few	2	3	3 – 4
Diencephalon	0 – few	1	2	3 – 4	4 – 5
Cerebral cortex	0	few – 2	1 – 2	1 – 3	2 – 4
Striatum	islands	islands	islands and diffuse	diffuse	diffuse

The density of catecholaminergic terminals in the various regions of the rat brain during development was determined by histofluorescent microscopy. Results are expressed in terms of a 0 to 5 scale. Adapted from Loizou (1972).

spective neurotransmitter that are anatomically, kinetically, and pharmacologically distinct (Coyle and Snyder, 1969; Horn et al., 1971). The noradrenergic neurons exhibit a saturable uptake for L-norepinephrine with a Km of 3×10^{-7} M, that is markedly sensitive to inhibition by the antidepressant, desipramine (Snyder and Coyle, 1969).

In the various regions of the adult brain, the synaptosomal uptake of norepinephrine is proportional to the density of innervation by noradrenergic terminals, and destruction of the terminals with 6-hydroxydopamine markedly reduces this uptake process (Snyder and Coyle, 1969; Uretsky and Iversen, 1970). Studies of the ontogenesis of the peripheral sympathetic nervous system indicate that the development of an organ's ability to take up norepinephrine parallels the development of its sympathetic innervation (Glowinski et al., 1964; Sachs et al., 1970). Therefore, analysis of the uptake of norepinephrine into synaptosomes should be a method for quantifying the increase in noradrenergic terminals in the developing brain.

In homogenates prepared from whole rat brain, the high-affinity uptake mechanism for norepinephrine appears at 18 days of gestation (Coyle and Axelrod, 1971). During subsequent maturation, the affinity constant (Km) does not change significantly, whereas the capacity to take up norepinephrine (V_{max}) increases over 100-fold for the whole brain. That this uptake process indeed represents the one specific for norepinephrine is substantiated by the fact that the inhibitory effect of desipramine shows a similar developmental profile.

The ^{3}H-norepinephrine accumulated by homogenates of adult brain is localized in the synaptosomal fractions on continuous sucrose gradients (Coyle and Snyder, 1969). This particulate-bound peak of ^{3}H-norepinephrine coincides with the peak of occluded lactic dehydrogenase activity, a more general enzymatic marker for synaptosomes, and occurs at a distinctly lower sucrose molarity than the peak of monoamine oxidase activity, an enzymatic marker for mitochondria (Figure 1). Analysis of the subcellular distribution of ^{3}H-norepinephrine accumulated by homogenates prepared from rat brains of different ages indicates that there is a progressive increase with age in the amount of ^{3}H-norepinephrine that sediments in the synaptosomal fractions. When corrected for brain weight, the real increase in the amount of synaptosomal-bound ^{3}H-norepinephrine is nearly 300-fold between 18 days of gestation and adulthood. The parallel increase in the specific uptake mechanism for norepinephrine and in the amount of synaptosomal-bound ^{3}H-norepinephrine suggest that uptake may be a valid index of the outgrowth of the noradrenergic terminals in the central nervous system.

Enzymes involved in the biosynthesis of catecholamines

The dopaminergic and noradrenergic neurons have in common the first two enzymes in the biosynthetic pathway for their neurotransmitters, tyrosine hydroxylase and dopa decarboxylase (Molinoff and Axelrod, 1971). The noradrenergic neurons possess an additional enzyme, dopamine-β-hydroxylase, which converts dopamine to norepinephrine. All three enzymes are present in the fetal rat brain at 15 days of gestation. During subsequent development, the activities of these enzymes increase 500-fold in the whole brain (Coyle and Axelrod, 1972a, 1972b; Lamprecht and Coyle, 1972; Figure 2). Thus, in confirmation of the observation made with the histofluorescent technique (Maeda and Dresse, 1969), the rat brain is capable of synthesizing catecholamines extremely early in ontogenesis. Furthermore, regression of enzyme activity back to zero suggests that these enzymes would first appear at 13 to 14 days of gestation. This coincides closely with the date established by the autoradiographic study as the time when differentiation of the noradrenergic neurons would commence.

Since the proliferating axons and terminals in the developing rat brain are identified by their catecholamine-induced fluorescence, it would appear likely that they also contain the enzymatic machinery necessary for the synthesis of the amines. Thus, the biosynthetic enzymes could be used as specific enzymatic markers for the outgrowth of the neuronal processes. The cell bodies of the noradrenergic neurons, which are located exclusively in the medulla-pons, send out processes that provide the noradrenergic innervation for the rest of the brain. In the fetal brain, dopamine-β-hydroxylase, the final enzyme in the synthesis pathway for norepinephrine, is localized primarily in the medulla-pons. With maturation, there is a progressive shift in enzyme activity to the rostral regions of the brain, so that by adulthood the medulla-pons possesses only 20% of the whole brain dopamine-β-hydroxylase activity (Coyle and Axelrod, 1972a). In the case of tyrosine hydroxylase, there is a 50% increase in its specific activity in the medulla-pons between birth and adulthood, whereas the cerebral cortex exhibits a sixfold increase in specific activity during the same period (Figure 3). The dopaminergic cell bodies that are located in the midbrain give rise to an extremely dense meshwork of terminals in the corpus striatum. During postnatal development, the specific activity of tyrosine hydroxylase in the midbrain increases only moderately in contrast to a 12-fold increase in the corpus striatum (Coyle and Axelrod, 1972b). Thus, with maturation, there is a centrifugal movement of the enzymes involved in the biosynthesis of catecholamines away from the regions of the brain that

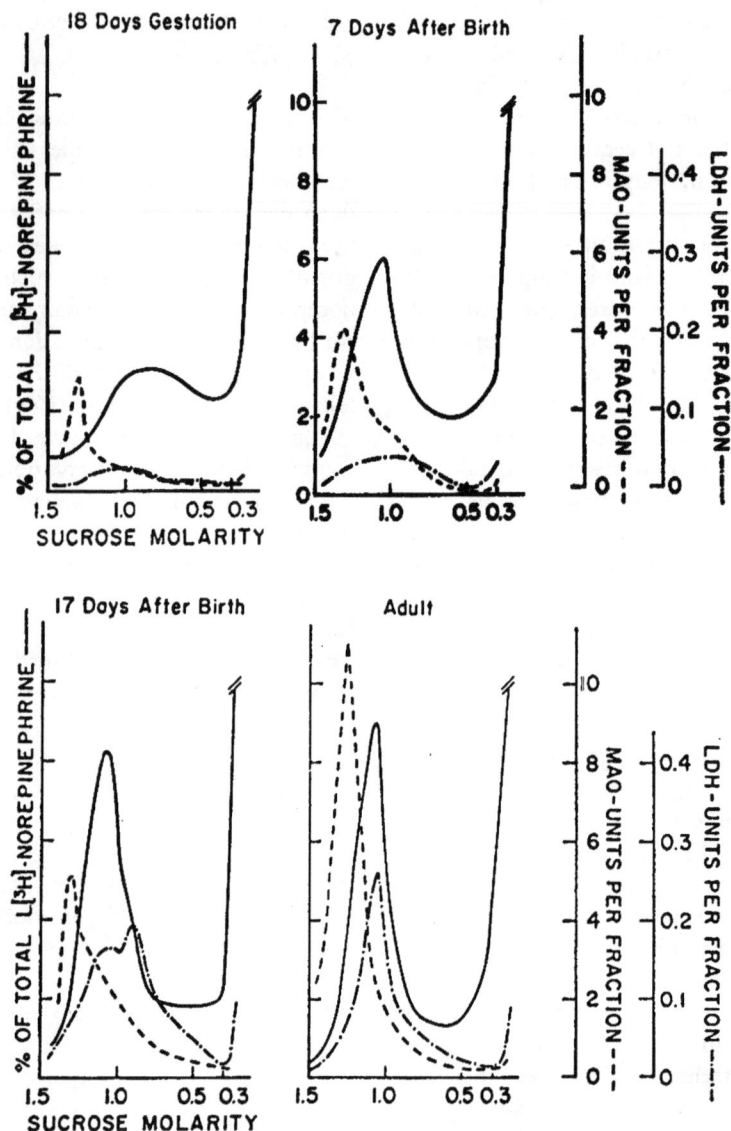

FIGURE 1 Sedimentation characteristics of L-[³H]norepinephrine, lactic dehydrogenase (LDH) and monoamine oxidase (MAO) in homogenates prepared from rat brains at various stages of development. The homogenates were incubated for 5 min with L-[³H]norepinephrine and the amount equivalent to 125 mg of brain tissue was centrifuged at 100,000 g on linear sucrose gradients (1.5 to 0.3 M). Total amount (nanomoles) of L-[³H]norepinephrine on the gradients were: 0.84 at 18 days of gestation; 2.47 at 7 days after birth; 3.07 at 17 days after birth; and 4.45 for the adult (adapted from Coyle and Axelrod, 1971).

contain the cell bodies to the regions that receive the terminals.

The temporal-spatial changes in enzyme activity during development are accompanied by changes in their subcellular distribution. For example, tyrosine hydroxylase in the adult rat brain behaves as a soluble enzyme, because it is released in the supernatant with the cytosol when the brain is homogenized in hypotonic buffer (Coyle, 1972). However, when the adult brain is homogenized in isotonic sucrose and fractionated according to the method of Whittaker (1965), most of the tyrosine hydroxylase is entrapped in and sediments with the synaptosomes, indicating a high degree of localization in the nerve terminals (Coyle, 1972; Figure 4). When fetal brain is fractionated in the same manner, most of the tyrosine hydroxylase is released into the supernatant, suggesting a nonterminal localization of the enzyme in the immature neuron. With age, there is a progressive redistribution of the enzyme from a soluble to a synaptosomal form (Coyle and Axelrod, 1972b). This regional and subcellular translocation of enzyme activity during development corresponds closely with the outgrowth of

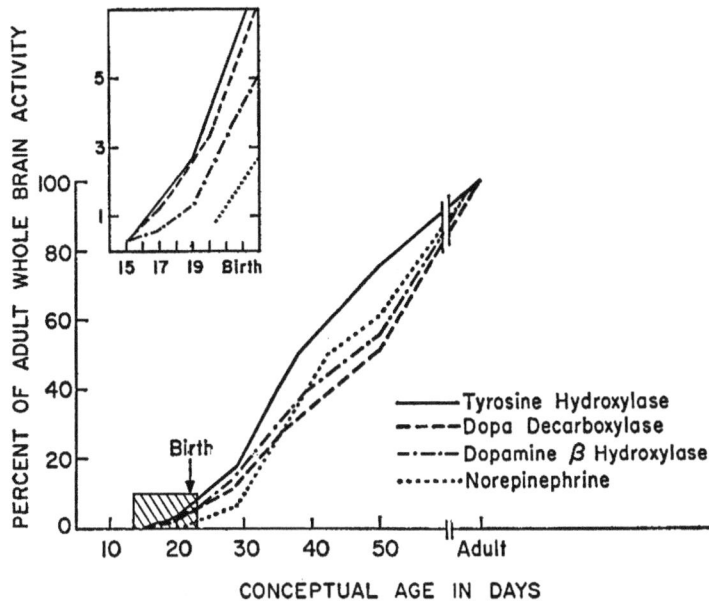

FIGURE 2 The development of total activity per brain of tyrosine hydroxylase, dopa decarboxylase, and dopamine-β-hydroxylase and total content of norepinephrine. Values are expressed in terms of percentage of whole brain activity for the adult rat.

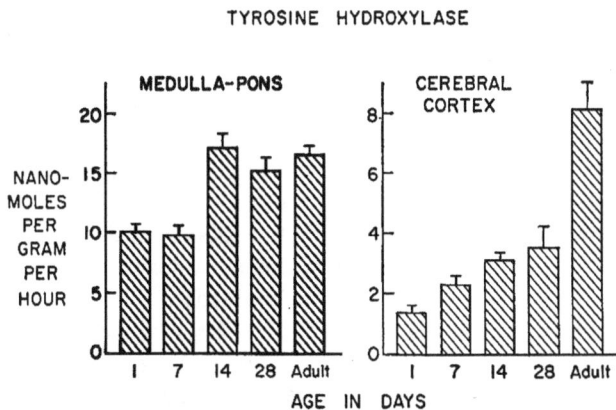

FIGURE 3 Changes in the specific activity of tyrosine hydroxylase in the medulla-pons and cerebral cortex of the rat brain during postnatal development (adapted from Coyle and Axelrod, 1972b).

the catecholaminergic processes as demonstrated by the histofluorescent technique.

An important distinction must be made between the density of innervation and the total amount of terminals in a particular region. This issue is especially relevant in the case of the cerebellum, a region that develops primarily after birth. The specific activities of both tyrosine hydroxylase and dopamine-β-hydroxylase increase about twofold between birth and adulthood in the cerebellum, which suggests only a small change in the density of noradrenergic innervation. However, the weight of the

cerebellum increases 35-fold during the same period. Therefore, the real increase in enzymatic activity and presumably the number of noradrenergic terminals in the cerebellum is in the order of 70-fold.

Functional characteristics of the differentiating neuron

Pharmacologic manipulation of the neurons in vivo can provide information about their functional characteristics. By means of an extremely sensitive enzymatic assay for norepinephrine (Henry and Coyle, in preparation), it has been possible to examine the effect of various pharmacologic agents on the disposition of the endogenous norepinephrine in the brain of the fetal rat at 18 days of gestation. At this stage, the brain has only 0.5% of the adult level of norepinephrine (Table II). Reserpine, a drug that inactivates the aminergic vesicular storage mechanism, causes a profound depletion of endogenous norepineprhine. Thus, vesicular storage plays a major role in protecting the transmitter from enzymatic degradation in the immature neuron. Inhibition of monoamine oxidase, the enzyme responsible for the intraneuronal catabolism of the catecholamines, or the administration of a large dose of the precursor, L-dopa, result in significant increases in the levels of norepinephrine. Inhibition of the initial enzyme in the biosynthetic pathway, tyrosine hydroxylase, with α-methyl-para-tyrosine causes a 50% depletion of norepinephrine

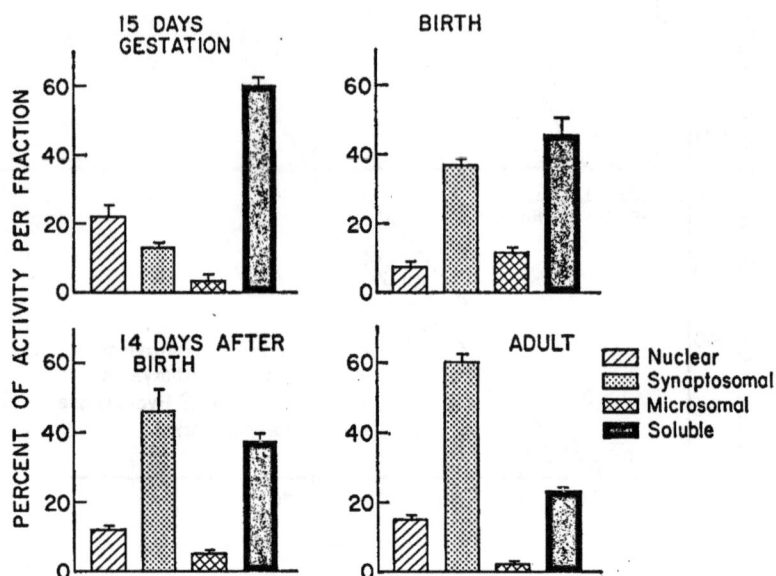

FIGURE 4 Distribution of tyrosine hydroxylase activity in subcellular fractions of rat brain during development. Subcellular fractions prepared from whole rat brains according to the method of Whittaker (1965) were assayed for tyrosine hydroxylase activity. The results are expressed as percentage of total recovered activity in each fraction.

TABLE II

Regulation of norepinephrine in rat brain at 18 days of gestation

Treatment	N	Percent of Control
Control	8	100 ± 8
Inhibition of storage (reserpine)	7	8 ± 2
Inhibition of tyrosine hydroxylase (α-methyl para tyrosine)	8	53 ± 3
Inhibition of monoamine oxidase (pheniprazine)	8	144 ± 8
L-Dopa and peripheral decarboxylase inhibitor	6	159 ± 22

Pregnant female rats were treated with drugs 3 to 5 hr prior to the removal of fetal brains. Norepinephrine content of control brains was 41 ± 4 picogram/milligram or 3.8 ± 0.4 nanogram/brain (Henry and Coyle, in preparation).

3 hours after treatment. This indicates a half-life for norepinephrine of approximately 3 hours, which is quite similar to that observed in the adult brain. In essence, the relative effects of these agents on the transmitter levels of the immature neurons are practically indistinguishable from those known to occur in the adult brain.

The fact that inhibition of tyrosine hydroxylase in the fetal rat causes a significant depletion of norepinephrine in the brain suggests that the central catecholaminergic neurons may be releasing neurotransmitter well before the completion of morphologic differentiation. The following studies lend support to this viewpoint: Amphet-

amine induces hyperactive and stereotypic behavior by releasing presynaptic catecholamines resulting in overstimulation of the postsynaptic receptors. Hyperactive and stereotypic behavior can be induced by amphetamine in the neonatal rat; in contrast, the inhibitory effect of the cholinergic neurons becomes operational 3 to 4 weeks later (Fibiger et al., 1970; McGeer et al., 1971). As early as 8 days after birth, there is a diurnal rhythm in the levels of endogenous norepinephrine in the rat brain with a peak in periods of darkness, which indicates a cyclic variation in the turnover of norepinephrine (Asano, 1971). Thus, the central catecholaminergic neurons appear to be physiologically functional well before they have become anatomically and biochemically fully developed.

Possible factors controlling development

Although there is currently little information concerning the factors that control the differentiation of the central catecholaminergic neurons, recent findings suggest a number of possibilities that merit further investigation. In the ontogenesis of the peripheral sympathetic ganglia of the chick, the neural crest cells give rise to catecholaminergic ganglioblasts in response to conditions imposed while the cells migrate ventrally; if this relationship is disturbed, the sympathoblasts fail to develop (Cohen, 1972). Similar intercellular interactions may occur when the nascent locus coeruleus migrates from its origin in the tegmentum. The biochemical development of the superior cervical ganglion of the mouse is, at least in part, controlled by the preganglionic cholinergic innervation (Black et al., 1971). In light of the developmental changes in the cholinesterase staining of the locus coeruleus (Maeda and Gerebtzoff, 1969), this mode of regulation appears tenable for certain central catecholaminergic neurons. An insulin-like hormone, nerve growth factor, plays an important, although poorly defined, role in the differentiation of the peripheral sympathetic neurons (Frazier et al., 1972). Since nerve growth factor stimulates axonal sprouting of sectioned central noradrenergic neurons (Björklund and Stenevi, 1972), it may also act as a trophic factor in the developing central nervous system.

Summary

Histologic and autoradiographic studies indicate that the major nuclei of the catecholaminergic neurons are formed well before birth in the rat brain. The outgrowth of the catecholaminergic axons and terminals occurs primarily during the 4 weeks after birth. During this period, there is a marked increase in the whole brain in the activity of the specific uptake mechanism for norepinephrine, a process associated with nerve terminals, as well as in the activity of the enzymes involved in the biosynthesis of catecholamines. Concurrently, there is a centrifugal movement of these enzymes from the regions of the brain that contain the cell bodies to the regions that receive the terminals. Indirect evidence suggests that the neurons may be physiologically functional well before the completion of morphologic and biochemical differentiation.

REFERENCES

AGRAWAL, H. C., S. N. GLISSON, and W. A. HIMWICH, 1968. Changes in monoamines of rat brain during postnatal ontogeny. *Biochim. Biophys. Acta* 130:511–513.

ALTMAN, J., 1966. Autoradiographic and histological studies of postnatal neurogenesis. I. A longitudinal investigation of the kinetics, migration and transformation of cells incorporating tritiated thymidine in neonatal rats, with special reference to postnatal neurogenesis in some brain regions. *J. Comp. Neurol.* 126:337–390.

ASANO, T., 1971. The maturation of the circadian rhythm of brain norepinephrine and 5-hydroxytryptamine in the rat. *Life Sci.* 10:883–894.

AXELROD, J., 1965. The metabolism, storage, and release of catecholamines. *Recent Prog. Hormone Res.* 21:597–622.

BJÖRKLUND, A., and V. STENEVI, 1972. Nerve growth factor: stimulation of regenerative growth of central noradrenergic neurons. *Science* 175:1251–1253.

BLACK, I. B., I. A. HENDRY, and L. L. IVERSEN, 1971. Trans-synaptic regulation of growth and development of adrenergic neurons in a mouse sympathetic ganglion. *Brain Res.* 34:229–240.

BREESE, G. R., and T. D. TRAYLOR, 1972. Developmental characteristics of brain catecholamines and tyrosine hydroxylase in the rat: effects of 6-hydroxydopamine. *Brit. J. Pharmacol.* 44:210–222.

COHEN, A. M., 1972. Factors directing the expression of sympathetic nerve traits in cells of neural crest origin. *J. Exp. Zool.* 179:167–182.

COYLE, J. T., 1972. Tyrosine hydroxylase in rat brain: cofactor requirements, regional and subcellular distribution. *Biochem. Pharmacol.* 21:1935–1944.

COYLE, J. T., and J. AXELROD, 1971. Development of the uptake and storage of L-[^{3}H]norepinephrine in the rat brain. *J. Neurochem.* 18:2061–2075.

COYLE, J. T., and J. AXELROD, 1972a. Dopamine-β-hydroxylase in the rat brain: developmental characteristics. *J. Neurochem.* 19:449–459.

COYLE, J. T., and J. AXELROD, 1972b. Tyrosine hydroxylase in rat brain: developmental characteristics. *J. Neurochem.* 19:1117–1123.

COYLE, J. T., and S. H. SNYDER, 1969. Catecholamine uptake by synaptosomes in homogenates of rat brain: stereospecificity in different areas. *J. Pharmacol. Exp. Ther.* 170:221–231.

DAVIS, J. M., F. K. GOODWIN, W. E. BUNNEY, D. L. MURPHY, and R. W. COLBURN, 1967. Effects of ions on uptake of norepinephrine by synaptosomes. *Pharmacologist* 9:184.

FALCK, B., and N.-A. HILLARP, 1959. On the cellular localization of catecholamines in the brain. *Acta Anat.* 38:277–279.

FIBIGER, H. C., L. D. LYTLE, and B. A. CAMPBELL, 1970. Cholinergic modulation of adrenergic arousal in the developing rat. *J. Comp. Phys. Psych.* 72:384–389.

FRAZIER, W. A., R. H. ANGELETTI, and R. A. BRADSHAW, 1972. Nerve growth factor and insulin. *Science* 176:482–488.

FUXE, K., T. HOKFELT, and U. UNGERSTEDT, 1970. Morphological and functional aspects of central monoamine neurons. *Inter. Rev. Neurobiol.* 13:93–126.

GLOWINSKI, J., J. AXELROD, I. J. KOPIN, and R. J. WURTMAN, 1964. Physiological disposition of ^{3}H-norepinephrine in the developing rat. *J. Pharmacol. Exp. Ther.* 146:48–53.

HORN, A. S., J. T. COYLE, and S. H. SNYDER, 1971. Catecholamine uptake by synaptosomes from rat brain. Structure-activity relationships of drugs with differential effects on dopamine and norepinephrine neurons. *Molec. Pharmacol.* 7:66–80.

JACOBSON, M., 1970. *Developmental Neurobiology.* New York: Holt, Rinehart and Winston.

LAMPRECHT, F., and J. T. COYLE, 1972. Dopa decarboxylase in the developing rat brain. *Brain Res.* 21:503–506.

LOIZOU, L. A., 1971. The postnatal development of monoamine-containing structures in the hypothalamo-hypophyseal system of the albino rat. *Z. Zellforsch.* 114:234–253.

LOIZOU, L. A., 1972. The postnatal ontogeny of monoamine-containing neurons in the central nervous system of the albino rat. *Brain Res.* 40:395–418.

LOIZOU, L. A., and P. SALT, 1970. Regional changes in monoamines of the rat brain during postnatal development. *Brain Res.* 20:467–470.

MAEDA, T., and A. DRESSE, 1969. Recherches sur le développment du locus coeruleus. 1. Etude des catécholamines au microscope de fluorescence. *Acta Neurol. Belg.* 69:5–10.

MAEDA, T., and M. A. GEREBTZOFF, 1969. Recherches sur le développment du locus coeruleus. 2. Etude histoenzymologique. *Acta Neurol. Belg.* 69:11–19.

McGEER, E. G., H. C. FIBIGER, and V. WICKSON, 1971. Differential development of caudate enzymes in the neonatal rat. *Brain Res.* 32:433–440.

MOLINOFF, P., and J. AXELROD, 1971. Biochemistry of catecholamines. *Ann. Rev. Biochem.* 40:465–500.

SACHS, C., J. DeCHAMPLAIN, T. MALMFORS, and L. OLSON, 1970. The postnatal development of noradrenaline uptake in the adrenergic nerves of different tissues from the rat. *Europ. J. Pharmacol.* 9:67–79.

SMITH, G. C., and R. W. SIMPSON, 1970. Monoamine fluorescence in the median eminence of foetal, neonatal and adult rats. *Z. Zellforsch.* 104:541–556.

SNYDER, S. H., and J. T. COYLE, 1969. Regional differences in ³H-norepinephrine and ³H-dopamine uptake into rat brain homogenates. *J. Pharmacol. Exp. Ther.* 165:78–86.

TISSARI, A. H., P. S. SCHÖNHÖFER, D. F. BOGDANSKI, and B. B.
BRODIE, 1969. Mechanism of biogenic amine transport II. Relationship between sodium and mechanism of ouabain blockade of the accumulation of serotonin and norepinephrine by synaptosomes. *Molec. Pharmacol.* 5:593–604.

UNGERSTEDT, U., 1971. Stereotaxic mapping of the monoamine pathways in the rat brain. *Acta Physiol. Scand.* Suppl. 367:1–48.

URETSKY, N. J., and L. L. IVERSEN, 1970. Effects of 6-hydroxy-dopamine on catecholamine containing neurons in the rat brain. *J. Neurochem.* 17:269–278.

WHITE, T. D., and P. KEEN, 1970. The role of internal and external Na⁺ and K⁺ on the uptake of [³H] noradrenalin by synaptosomes prepared from rat brain. *Biochim. Biophys. Acta* 196:285–295.

WHITTAKER, V. P., 1965. The application of subcellular fractionation techniques to the study of brain function. *Progr. Biophys. Molec. Biol.* 15:39–96.

78 Changes in Enzyme Activities in Neural Tissues with Maturation and Development of the Nervous System

LOUIS SOKOLOFF

ABSTRACT The brain of most mammalian species is largely undeveloped at birth and undergoes a major portion of its morphological, biochemical, and functional maturation in early postnatal life. A number of enzyme activities related to energy metabolism show characteristic developmental profiles during this period of life. One mitochondrial enzyme, D-β-hydroxybutyrate dehydrogenase (HOBDH), which is involved in ketone body utilization, exhibits a particularly unique pattern of postnatal development in the brain. Along with other mitochondrial enzymes of energy metabolism, it is low at birth and rises during the nursing period to a maximum level. In contrast to the other enzymes, however, that maintain their maximum activities through adult life, HOBDH begins to decline after weaning, until it falls to relatively low levels in adulthood. A similar pattern is exhibited by 3-ketoacid transferase, the second enzyme in the pathway of ketone body utilization. The changes in the activities of these two enzymes follow the level of ketosis in the blood and allow the brain, which normally utilizes glucose almost exclusively as its substrate, to adapt its substrate utilization to the availability of ketone bodies in the blood. The changes in the level of HOBDH in brain during development appear to be, at least in part, regulated by nutritional and hormonal factors.

THE MULTIPLICITY of biochemical processes proceeding in the tissues at all times necessitates the operation of control mechanisms to coordinate, adjust, or adapt the pattern of metabolic activities to the continually changing needs of the cell. The central theme of all the preceding presentations in this part has been that such control is achieved mainly by regulation of the levels or behavior of protein molecules, particularly those with enzyme functions. Indeed, it is a truism that, although the information for life is encoded in the molecular structure of nucleic acids, the translation of this information into actual life processes is accomplished only through the mediation of proteins. Proteins are major constituents of all the structural elements and comprise almost the entire catalytic apparatus of the cell. As emphasized by Schimke, earlier in this part, all proteins, structural, functional, and enzymatic, are in a constant state of turnover. Their turnover rates are markedly individualized and diverse and vary with the physiological state and special circumstances of the cell. The amount of any given protein present is determined by the net balance of its rates of synthesis and degradation. In almost all cases that have been examined, proteins are synthesized at a constant rate and degraded exponentially; the steady-state level of each protein is, therefore, determined by the ratio of its zero-order rate of synthesis to its first-order rate constant of degradation (Schimke, 1969). The level of any protein can, therefore, be altered by modification of its rate of synthesis, its rate constant of degradation, or both. Since biochemical reactions are generally proportional to the concentrations of the enzymatic proteins that catalyze them, control of enzyme levels through adjustment of their rates of synthesis or degradation constitutes one of the most important mechanisms of biochemical regulation in the tissues.

Enzymes are macromolecular catalysts and as such facilitate the chemical interconversions of the many small molecules that comprise the substance of metabolism. The rates of the reactions that they catalyze are determined not merely by the concentrations of the enzymes and their substrates but also by their catalytic efficiency and effectiveness. It has become apparent in recent years that enzymes are not simply passive catalysts, like iron filings or platinum black, but are dynamic elements with readily modifiable, three-dimensional structures that markedly influence their binding affinities for the substrates and their catalytic efficiency. The conformation and, therefore, catalytic activity of an enzyme molecule can vary with the nature of the intracellular environment in which it finds itself. In addition to the general environmental conditions, such as temperature, pH, and ionic strength, there are specific mechanisms for conformational control. These usually involve the binding of small molecules to specific binding sites in the enzyme. It has long been known that enzymes have specific binding sites

LOUIS SOKOLOFF National Institute of Mental Health, Bethesda, Maryland for their substrates; the concentrations of the substrates regulate the enzyme activity in relation to the degree of saturation of these binding sites. This phenomenon is quantitatively described in the Michaelis-Menten relationship. However, for many enzymes, there are other binding sites, specific either for substrate or other small molecules, that are not catalytic but regulatory; the binding of the specific ligand to these sites does not serve the catalytic process directly but results in modification of the enzyme's conformation so as to alter its affinity for its substrate or its catalytic efficiency. Catalytic activity may be positively or negatively affected. The conformational change may be relatively simple and involve only a spatial reorientation of an otherwise unchanged species of protein, or, in the case of multimeric enzymes, there may be a dissociation of the enzyme into its component subunits or the converse. The nature and mechanisms of allosteric regulation of enzyme activity have been comprehensively reviewed by Koshland (1970). The essential point for consideration at present is that biochemical regulation can be achieved not only by changes in the levels of enzymes but also by control of the catalytic activity of already existing enzyme molecules.

These basic mechanisms of biochemical regulation operate in all tissues including those of the central nervous system. Their influences permeate throughout almost all biochemical processes and are manifested in the brain throughout the entire life span. Previous notions that the fully mature brain is biochemically fixed, rigid, and inflexible have yielded to accumulating evidence that it retains the capability to undergo metabolic adaptations to changing needs and circumstances and enjoys biochemical as well as structural and functional plasticity (McIlwain, 1971). It has long been obvious, of course, that the orderly, coordinated sequence of changes that characterize the postnatal development of the brain is only the expression of an exquisitely organized, controlled, and regulated program of biochemical events. It is probably fair to say that in no case have the relative contributions of the various potential mechanisms for biochemical regulation to the changes seen in brain been sorted out and definitely established, but their operation and their value to the maintenance of the structural and functional integrity of the organ are clearly discernible. It is beyond the scope of this book to cover comprehensively the variety of manifestations of biochemical regulation in the nervous system. Axelrod and Coyle, respectively, in previous chapters, have presented examples in the area of neurotransmitter biochemistry. In the remainder of this chapter, we shall concern ourselves with other examples, particularly in relation to the processes of energy metabolism and their regulation during postnatal maturation of the brain.

General features of postnatal maturation of the brain

The brain of most mammalian species, including man, is largely underdeveloped at birth and undergoes a major portion of its morphological, functional, and biochemical maturation in early postnatal life. Postnatal maturation does not merely represent growth but continued differentiation. The changes that occur are so extensive that essentially a transformation into a phenotypically different organ is achieved. The process is comparable to that of amphibian metamorphosis in which the tadpole is ultimately converted into a frog. Interestingly enough, both the metamorphosis of the frog and the postnatal maturation of the brain are dependent on the presence of thyroid hormones, and in both cases sensitivity to these hormones is lost after complete maturation is achieved.

The postnatal morphogenesis and functional development of mammalian brain have been most extensively studied in the rat, mainly by Eayrs and his associates (Eayrs, 1964). In this species, maturation is achieved in the first 5 to 6 weeks of life after birth. Normally, the brain increases in size approximately 4- to 5-fold during this period, but the most dramatic changes are observed in the microscopic appearance of the tissue. The neurons increase in size, mainly because of an increase in perikaryonal cytoplasm. There is a marked proliferation of axonal and dendritic processes, and the density of axodendritic connections is strikingly increased, particularly in the neuropil. Myelin is laid down around the axons, and the nerve cell bodies become less densely packed because the spaces between them become filled with axonal and dendritic processes and myelin.

A number of physiological changes occur in parallel with the morphogenetic development. Innate reflexes, such as the startle, righting, and placing reactions that are absent at birth, appear at various times during the maturational period. Learning behavior, manifested by conditioned reflex activity, appears. The electroencephalogram, which is slow and low in amplitude at birth, speeds up and increases in voltage. Evoked potential responses make their appearance and then develop shorter latencies, higher amplitudes, and shorter duration.

The morphological and functional changes are accompanied by extensive biochemical changes (Sokoloff, 1971). Some of these changes reflect the altered morphological state of the tissues, i.e., the less dense packing of cells and the growth and expansion of the perikaryonal cytoplasm. Others result from continued postnatal differentiation. Protein and RNA concentrations and contents increase as the water content decreases and the perikaryonal cytoplasm enlarges. Cell proliferation proceeds for only a short time after birth, but thereafter the nuclei do not increase very significantly in size and amount; the DNA concentration, therefore, falls as the constant amount of DNA becomes diluted by the increasing cytoplasmic mass and myelin. Lipid composition is radically altered and reflects to a large extent the deposition of myelin.

That biochemical regulatory mechanisms underlie the maturational process is evidenced by the extensive realignment of enzyme patterns that occurs during this period. An impressive number of enzyme activities are altered during maturation. Table I presents only a partial list of those enzymes that have been found to change in activity during maturation of the brain. Increasing activity is the usual pattern though not common to all enzymes, indicating that the developmental process is selective and specific. A few enzyme activities decline again after the initial increase; others do not change at all; and some decline during the maturational process.

As previously noted, the postnatal development of the brain is largely controlled by the thyroid hormones. If the animal is thyroidectomized at birth, then many of the morphological, functional, and biochemical changes associated with maturation are retarded or prevented, and the brain never develops normal structure and function. Thyroid hormone replacement therapy allows these changes to progress normally, provided that it is initiated early enough. In the rat the critical period appears to be the first 24 days of life (Eayrs, 1964). The earlier the initiation of therapy, the more complete and normal is the development of the brain, but if begun after 24 days of age, thyroid hormone administration has little beneficial effect on brain development. Indeed, it is well known that in the adult, normal or cretinous, the brain is incapable of direct response to thyroid hormones (Eayrs, 1964; Sokoloff, 1971).

The mechanism of action of thyroid hormones remains undefined, but almost certainly their role in the development of the brain reflects to a large extent their ability to stimulate protein and RNA synthesis (Sokoloff and Kaufman, 1961; Tata and Widnell, 1966). Thyroid hormones stimulate protein synthesis in brain only

TABLE I

Some enzyme activities reported to change during postnatal maturation of the brain

Enzyme	Direction of Change	References
Hexokinase	+	Schwark et al., 1972
Phosphofructokinase	+	Schwark et al., 1972
Aldolase	+	Hamburgh and Flexner, 1957; Swaiman et al., 1970
Pyruvic kinase	+	Schwark et al., 1972
Creatine kinase	+	Swaiman et al., 1970
NADP$^+$-isocitrate dehydrogenase	+	Murthy and Rappoport, 1963; Swaiman et al., 1970
Succinic dehydrogenase	+	Hamburgh and Flexner, 1957; Garcia Argiz et al., 1967
Cytochrome oxidase	+	Hamburgh and Flexner, 1957; Klee and Sokoloff, 1967
D-β-Hydroxybutyrate dehydrogenase	+ followed by −	Klee and Sokoloff, 1967; Krebs et al., 1971
3-Ketoacid transferase	+ followed by −	Krebs et al., 1971
Alanine aminotransferase	+	Balzsá et al., 1968
Aspartate aminotransferase	+	Pasquini et al., 1967
Aspartate carbamoyltransferase	−	Pasquini et al., 1967
Fatty acid synthetase	−	Volpe and Kishimoto, 1972
Cholinesterase	+	Hamburgh and Flexner, 1957
Tyrosine hydroxylase	+	Coyle, 1973
Dopa decarboxylase	+	Coyle, 1973
Dopamine-β-hydroxylase	+	Coyle, 1973
Glutamic decarboxylase	+	Garcia Argiz et al., 1967; Balzsá et al., 1968
GABA transaminase	+	Garcia Argiz et al., 1967
Na$^+$, K$^+$-ATPase	+	Garcia Argiz et al., 1967; Valcana and Timiras, 1969
Mg^{2+}-ATPase	+	Garcia Argiz et al., 1967; Valcana and Timiras, 1969
Adenyl cyclase	+	Schmidt and Robison, 1972
cAMP phosphodiesterase	+	Schmidt and Robison, 1972

during the period of its growth and development; they have no such effect in fully mature brain (Michels et al., 1963; Klee and Sokoloff, 1964; Sokoloff, 1971). Their effects on RNA and protein synthesis are themselves, however, secondary to an earlier metabolic change arising from a prior interaction between the hormones and the mitochondrial components of the cell (Sokoloff and Kaufman, 1961; Sokoloff et al., 1968; Sokoloff, 1968). The mitochondria appear to contain the locus of the primary biochemical action of the thyroid hormones (Sokoloff, 1968). Evidence has accumulated that indicates that mitochondria of immature brain share with mitochondria of other thyroxine-sensitive tissues the ability to participate with thyroxine in this prerequisite primary reaction, but in the course of development the mitochrondria of brain appear to lose this capacity (Klee and Sokoloff, 1964). It is a change in the properties of the mitochondria that appears to be the basis for the difference in thyroxine-sensitivities of immature and mature brain (Sokoloff, 1970).

Energy metabolism of the brain

CEREBRAL OXYGEN CONSUMPTION The transformation of the relatively poorly differentiated organ at birth into the enormously complex and elegantly performing apparatus that constitutes the mature brain is accompanied by a marked increase in its energy consumption. Cerebral oxygen consumption is low at birth and rises in a typical S-shaped growth-type of curve until it finally levels off in the mature brain at a level more than double that present at birth (Figure 1) (Fazekas et al., 1951). The thyroid hormones, which promote the postnatal maturation of the brain and may in small excess accelerate the process, shift the development pattern for oxidative metabolism to the left, causing an earlier and steeper rise and a more rapid achievement of the normal mature level; once the mature level is reached, however, the continued administration of thyroxine has no further effect on cerebral oxygen consumption (Figure 1).

The rate of oxygen utilization by the mature brain is among the highest of all tissues of the body. In normal conscious adult man, cerebral oxygen consumption equals approximately 3.5 ml per 100 g of tissue per minute or about 800 ml per minute for the entire brain, an energy expenditure of close to 20 watts (Kety, 1957; Sokoloff, 1972). The magnitude of this rate can be appreciated when one considers that the brain of adult man, which comprises only 2% of total body weight, alone consumes almost 20% of the total body basal oxygen consumption. The nature of the processes that consume this enormous amount of energy is not entirely clear. The brain does not do mechanical work like cardiac or skeletal muscle or

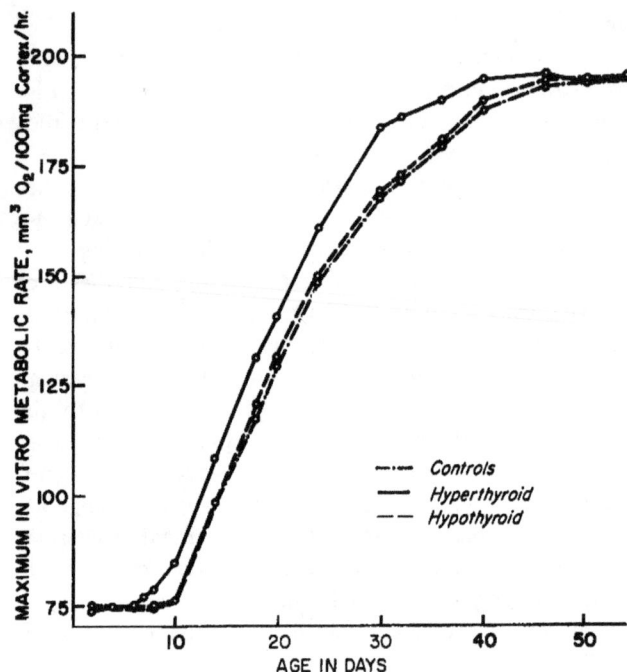

FIGURE 1 Changes in cerebral cortical oxygen consumption in rat brain during postnatal maturation and the influence of thyroid status on the developmental process. From Fazekas et al. (1951).

osmotic work like kidney. The mature brain does not have the complex energy-consuming metabolic and biosynthetic functions of liver. Clearly, the functions of nervous tissues are primarily excitation and conduction, and these are reflected in the unceasing electrical activity of the brain. The electrical energy is ultimately derived from chemical processes, and it is likely that most of the brain's energy consumption is utilized for active transport of ions to sustain and restore the membrane potentials discharged during the processes of excitation and conduction.

NORMAL SUBSTRATES OF CEREBRAL ENERGY METABOLISM The rapid rate of energy metabolism of the mature brain requires the continuous replenishment of its nutrient supply by the blood flow. In the mature brain under normal conditions, it appears that glucose is the almost exclusive substrate for its oxidative metabolism (Kety, 1957; Sokoloff, 1972). The rates of cerebral oxygen and glucose consumption in conscious, young adult man under physiological conditions are approximately 156 μmole and 31 μmole per 100 g of tissue per minute, respectively (Sokoloff, 1972). The CO_2 production is essentially equivalent to O_2 consumption, and the cerebral respiratory quotient (RQ) is, therefore, close to unity (Kety, 1957). An RQ of 1.0 indicates that the O_2 is consumed and the CO_2 produced in the oxidation of carbohydrate.

The O_2 consumption is equivalent to the amount required for the complete oxidation of 26 μmole of glucose to CO_2 and water. Since the measured steady-state rate of glucose consumption is 31 μmole/100 g/min, there is more than enough glucose consumed to account for all of the O_2 consumption. The excess glucose is probably distributed in various intermediates of carbohydrate metabolism, each of which is normally released into the blood in such small amounts as to be virtually undetectable in the arteriovenous differences. On the basis of cerebral arteriovenous differences, there appears to be under normal circumstances no steady-state uptake of any potential substrate for oxidative metabolism other than glucose in more than trivial amounts. The combination of a cerebral RQ of unity, an almost stoichiometric relationship between oxygen and glucose consumption, and the absence of any significant arteriovenous difference for any other potential substrate constitutes strong evidence that the adult brain derives its energy under normal conditions almost solely from the aerobic oxidation of glucose.

The fact that the brain normally consumes only glucose for energy does not distinguish between preferential and obligatory utilization of glucose. Most tissues are facultative in their choice of substrates and use them interchangeably in accordance with their availability from the blood. It was once believed that the brain did not enjoy such flexibility and was rigidly restricted to glucose for its substrate (Kety, 1957). This conviction was based on the obvious impairments of cerebral function and energy metabolism that occur when the brain is deprived of glucose and the inability of other potential substrates to substitute for glucose to prevent or reverse these effects.

Hypoglycemia is associated with changes in mental state, ranging from mild, subjective sensory disturbances to convulsions, coma, and death, depending on both the degree and duration of the hypoglycemia. The behavioral effects are accompanied by abnormalities in the electroencephalogram and cerebral metabolic rate, and cerebral oxygen consumption declines in proportion to the depression of the level of consciousness (Kety, 1957; Sokoloff, 1972). The cerebral effects of hypoglycemia are independent of the mode of its induction and are similar whether the hypoglycemia is caused by insulin or hepatic insufficiency (Kety, 1957). All the effects are prevented or rapidly reversed by glucose administration, provided that they have not been allowed to persist until irreversible changes have occurred. Many potential substrates have been tested for their ability to substitute for glucose and prevent or reverse the cerebral effects of hypoglycemia. Few have been found effective, and of these all but one appear to operate by raising the blood glucose level rather than by serving directly as a substrate for cerebral

metabolism (Sokoloff, 1972). Only mannose can be used directly or sufficiently rapidly by the brain to replace glucose and restore normal cerebral function, even in the complete absence of glucose (Sloviter and Kamimoto, 1970). It traverses the blood-brain barrier and is converted to mannose-6-phosphate by hexokinase, which phosphorylates mannose as effectively as glucose. Mannose-6-phosphate is then isomerized to fructose-6-phosphate by phosphomannoseisomerase, which is quite active in brain tissue (Kizer and McCoy, 1960). It is through this pathway that mannose replaces glucose and maintains an adequate glycolytic flux. Maltose produces arousal from insulin coma, but only by raising the blood glucose level through its conversion to glucose by maltase activity in blood and other tissues (Sloviter and Kamimoto, 1970; Sokoloff, 1972). Epinephrine is quite effective, but by stimulating hepatic glycogenolysis and consequently elevating blood glucose concentration. Glutamate, arginine, p-aminobenzoate, and succinate are also occasionally effective, but probably through the release of epinephrine which in turn raises the blood glucose level (Sokoloff, 1972). Many substances tested and found ineffective are compounds normally formed and utilized within the brain and are normal intermediates in its intermediary metabolism. Lactate, pyruvate, fructose-diphosphate, acetate, β-hydroxybutyrate, and acetoacetate are such examples (Kety, 1957; Sokoloff, 1972). These can all be utilized by brain slices, homogenates, or cell-free fractions, and the enzymes for their metabolism are present in brain. In some cases, as for example, glycerol (Sloviter et al., 1966, 1967) or ethanol (Raskin and Sokoloff, 1970), the enzymes may not be present in sufficient amounts to sustain the high rate of utilization required by the brain. In other cases, for example, acetoacetate and D-β-hydroxybutyrate (Krebs et al., 1971), the enzymes are adequate, but the substrate is insufficient because of inadequate blood level or restricted transport through the blood-brain barrier. The brain requires continuous delivery of substrate by the blood, and there is thus far no known endogenous substance present in blood in sufficient amounts to substitute fully for glucose as a substrate for cerebral energy metabolism. The one substance, mannose, which has been found to be a suitable replacement, is not a significant constituent of blood. Glucose must, therefore, be considered essential for the physiological and biochemical functioning of the nervous system.

Utilization of ketone bodies by the brain

The impressive mass of evidence accumulated over several decades pointing to glucose as the essential and almost exclusive substrate for cerebral energy metabolism led to the long-held belief that the brain was inflexible and uncompromising in its choice of nutrients. It is known, of course, that the brain is the mediator of a number of reflexes that regulate somatic functions to modify the distribution of blood flow and the composition of the blood in a manner advantageous to itself. The carotid sinus reflex, for example, clearly serves to maintain cerebral blood flow even at the expense of other less vital organs. Hypoglycemia and anoxia initiate sympathetic outflow and epinephrine release, which in turn maintain or enhance cerebral bood flow and the glucose content of the blood. It was, therefore, believed that the brain responds to extenuating circumstances not by intrinsic adaptation but by adjusting bodily functions to its needs through its reflex control of somatic physiological and metabolic processes. Recent evidence has forced a revision of this belief. It is now apparent that the brain, like most other tissues, is capable of metabolic adaptation (McIlwain, 1971), even with respect to its choice of substrates for energy metabolism (Krebs et al., 1971). Although there is still no convincing evidence that it can

function in the complete absence of glucose, the brain is now known to substitute other substrates, at least in part, for glucose in conditions in which these other substrates become more available and the glucose supply limited. The ketone bodies, D(-)-β-hydroxybutyrate and acetoacetate, are such substances, and the brain utilizes them in a variety of ketotic states in proportion, more or less, to their concentrations in blood. These ketone bodies, which are interconvertible into one another, are by-products of the metabolism of fatty acids (Figure 2). Their levels in blood are normally very low, but their rates of production are enhanced when fatty acid metabolism is increased, probably because the decrease in free CoA and the rise in acetyl CoA levels associated with accelerated fatty acid degradation shift the sequence of metabolic reactions in the direction of their formation (Figure 2). They are produced mainly in the liver, whichcan make them but cannot utilize them, because it lacks succinyl CoA: 3-oxoacid CoA-transferase (Mahler, 1953), the enzyme that converts free acetoacetate to acetoacetyl CoA, an essential step in the utilization of ketone bodies (Figure 2).

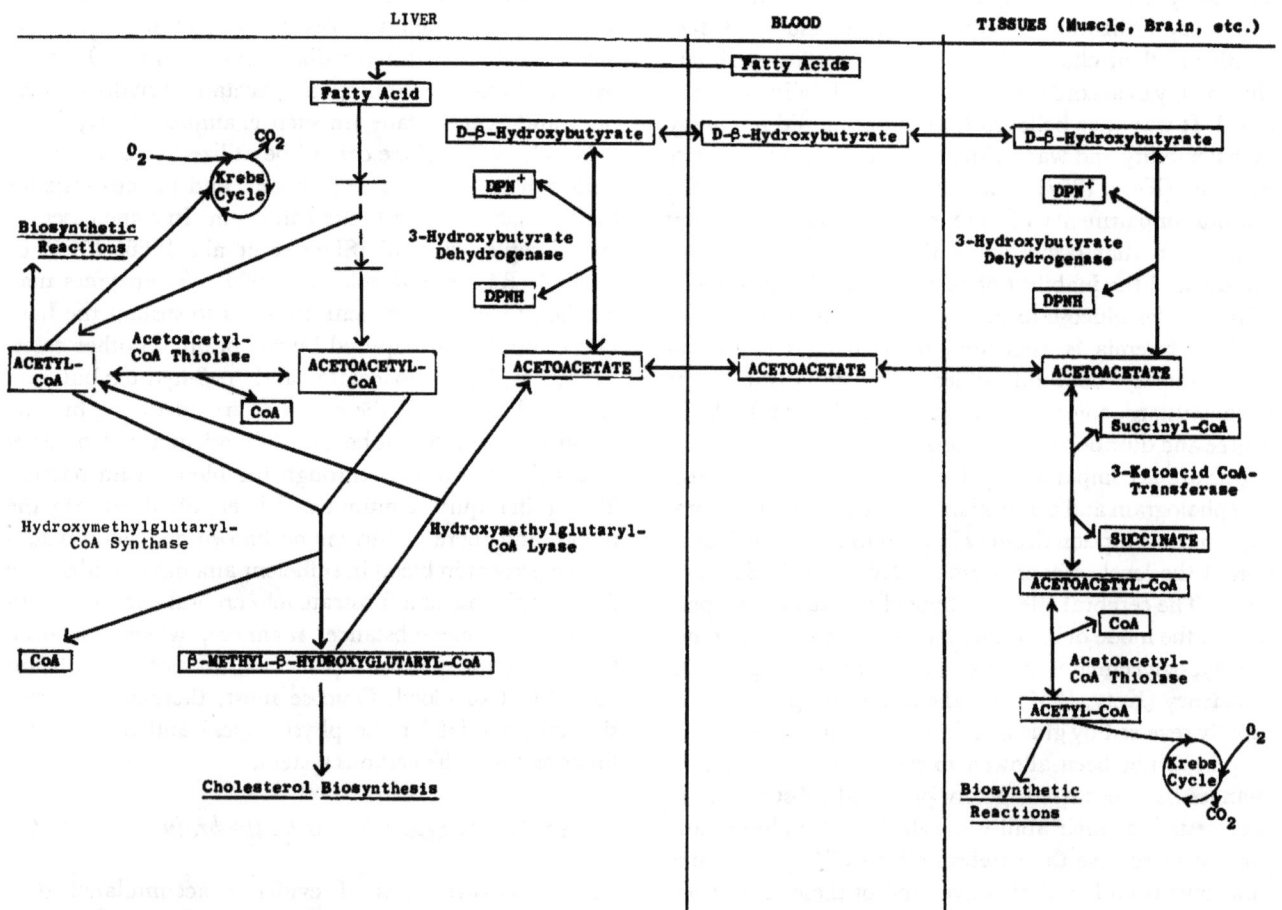

FIGURE 2   Metabolic pathways and enzymes of ketone body formation and utilization.

As the liver metabolizes fatty acids, it produces ketone bodies that are released into the blood and circulated for utilization by other tissues. Conditions in which fatty acid metabolism by liver is increased lead to elevated levels of ketone bodies in the blood.

STARVATION Evidence that the brain can extract and utilize ketone bodies from the blood was first obtained by Owen et al. (1967) in human subjects being treated for obesity by complete and prolonged starvation. The total body carbohydrate stores of the patients at the onset of the fast were estimated to be between 150 and 300 g, and metabolic balance studies indicated that their maximum rate of gluconeogenesis from protein and glycerol during the fast could not have exceeded 33 g per day. Since cerebral glucose utilization is normally approximately 110 g per day, the total body's actual and potential glucose reserves were clearly insufficient to satisfy the brain's normal glucose requirements for more than a few days. Nevertheless, after 6 to 7 weeks of starvation, these patients exhibited none of the usual signs of cerebral dysfunction indicative of cerebral glucose insufficiency. Their level of consciousness, EEG, and performance on psychometric testing remained within normal limits, evidence of adequate rates of cerebral energy metabolism despite the insufficiency of glucose to support it. Clearly the brain must have turned to the utilization of other substrates. The enigma of the nature of the substrate was resolved by examination of the cerebral arteriovenous differences (Table II). As expected, the glucose arteriovenous difference had declined to about half of its normal level, and of this, about half was accounted for by lactate and pyruvate release and did not, therefore, support oxidative metabolism. Net lactate and pyruvate production by brain is normally barely, if at all, detectable (Kety, 1957). The arteriovenous oxygen difference was normal, and glucose utilization, after correction for lactate and pyruvate recovery, accounted for only about 30% of it. Most of the remainder of the oxygen consumption was apparently supported by the ketone bodies, D-β-hydroxybutyrate and acetoacetate, which accounted for 52% and 8%, respectively. The remainder of the oxygen consumption could be accounted for by the uptake of α-amino nitrogen-containing material, presumably amino acids. No evidence of fatty acid utilization was observed. An ancillary finding of interest was the remarkably low cerebral RQ of 0.63. None of the substrates being oxidized could lead to so low an RQ, and it suggests that there is considerable CO_2 fixation and/or gluconeogenesis going on within the brain during starvation.

The changes in cerebral metabolism during starvation demonstrate that the mature brain is capable of adapting to altered nutrient supply. Normally it relies on glucose almost exclusively as the substrate for its energy metabolism, but availability of glucose becomes limited during starvation. On the other hand, starvation causes mobilization of fatty acids from the fat stores in adipose tissue, and the accelerated metabolism of fatty acids by liver leads in turn to enhanced formation of ketone bodies and the elevation of their levels in blood. The brain adapts to the altered conditions by switching in part from consumption of the endangered glucose supply to utilization of the ketone bodies made available by the alterations in body metabolism.

TABLE II

*Substrates of cerebral energy metabolism in human adults during prolonged starvation**

Substance	Arterial Concentration	Arteriovenous Differences		
		In Measured Units	Calculated O$_2$ Equivalent	
			(vol. %)	(μmole/ 100 ml)
Total glucose	449 μmole/100 ml (81 mg %)	26 μmole/100 ml (4.7 mg %)	—	—
Glucose (after correction for lactate and pyruvate)	—	14.5 μmole/100 ml (2.6 mg %)	2.0	88
β-Hydroxybutyrate†	667 μmole/100 ml	34 μmole/100 ml	3.4	153
Acetoacetate†	117 μmole/100 ml	6 μmole/100 ml	0.5	24
α-Amino nitrogen	314 μmole/100 ml	9 μmole/100 ml	0.9	42
Total Calculated O$_2$ Equivalents			6.8	307
Measured Arteriovenous O$_2$ Differences§			6.6	296

*From data of Owen et al. (1967).

†1 mole of β-hydroxybutyrate and acetoacetate equivalent to 4.5 and 4.0 moles of O_2, respectively.

§Measured cerebral respiratory quotient found to be 0.63.

INFANCY Like the human infant, the newborn rat is transiently hypoglycemic immediately after birth, and its blood ketone levels are also very low initially, as low as those of the normal fed adult rat (Krebs et al., 1971). With the onset of suckling, however, the blood ketone levels rise as much as 10-fold, and a true ketosis ensues (Figure 3) (Krebs et al., 1971). This ketosis is of nutritional origin; it reflects the ketogenic nature of maternal rat milk that contains 50% of its dry weight as fat (Dymsza et al., 1964). The ketosis persists throughout the suckling period until approximately 20 to 22 days of age when the rat is weaned onto a normal high-carbohydrate diet; the ketosis then gradually disappears and the blood ketone levels decline to the low levels characteristic of the well-nourished adult rat (Figure 3). During the ketosis of the suckling period, ketone bodies constitute an important source of the brain's substrates, and positive cerebral arteriovenous differences of D-β-hydroxybutyrate and acetoacetate proportional to their concentrations in the blood are observed (Figure 4) (Krebs et al., 1971; Hawkins et al., 1971). Similar evidence for significant cerebral ketone body utilization during normal infancy has been obtained in canine puppies (Spitzer and Weng, 1972) and human infants (Persson et al., 1972). Because the enzymes of ketone utilization in brain are more active in early postnatal life than in the adult, as will be discussed below, the brain of the infant is more efficient than the adult brain in extracting and utilizing ketone bodies from the blood at any given arterial concentration (Figure 4).

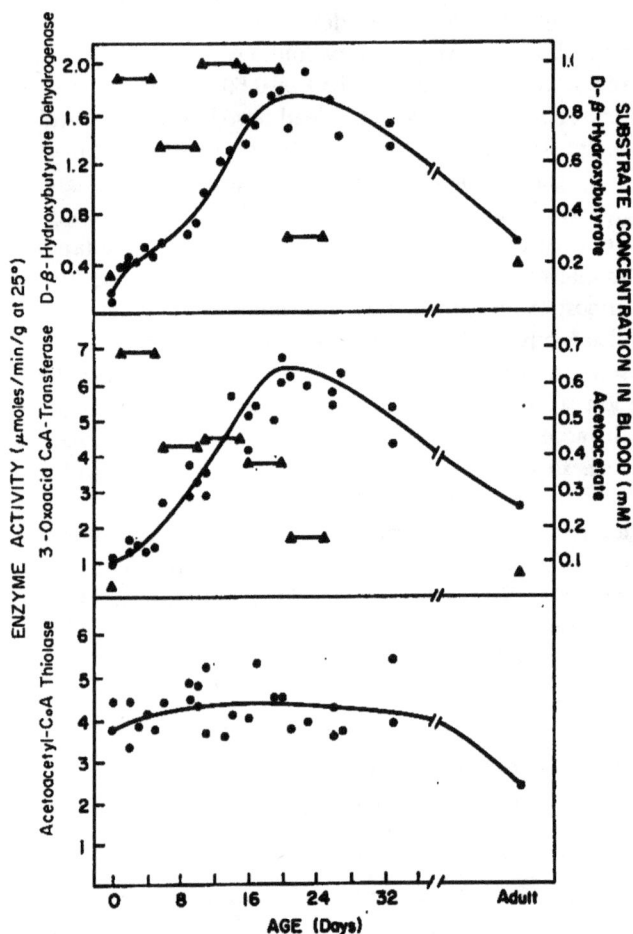

FIGURE 3 Changes in arterial blood levels of ketone bodies and the activities of the enzymes of ketone body utilization in the brain of the rat during postnatal maturation. Arterial ketone concentration, ▲——▲; enzyme activity in brain, ●——●. D-β-hydroxybutyrate dehydrogenase and acetoacetyl-CoA thiolase were assayed in the direction of ketone body utilization. The 3-oxoacid CoA-transferase (3-ketoacid transferase) was assayed in the reverse direction, the rate of which is approximately 5 times faster than that of the forward direction. For comparison of the rates of the enzymes all in the direction of ketone body utilization, the rates of the transferase activity presented in the figure should be divided by 5. (Illustration prepared from the data of Krebs et al., 1971.)

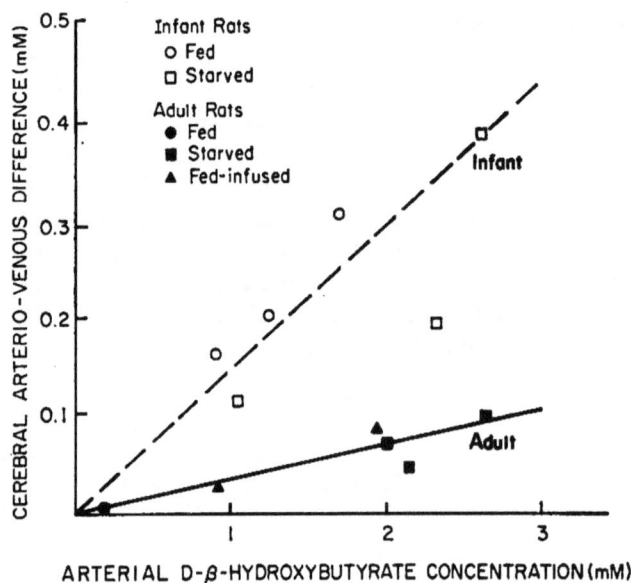

FIGURE 4 Influence of arterial concentrations on cerebral arteriovenous differences of ketone bodies in adult and infant rats. (Illustration composed of combination of figures from report of Krebs et al., 1971.)

MISCELLANEOUS KETOTIC STATES The brain can utilize D-β-hydroxybutyrate and acetoacetate whenever they are available but does not normally do so in adult life because of their low concentrations in the arterial blood. Ketosis of various origins can, therefore, lead to significant utilization of ketones by brain at any period of life. For example, fat feeding or the infusion of D-β-hydroxybutyrate or acetoacetate, which raises the blood levels of one or both ketone bodies, also leads to uptake of the ketones by brain in approximate proportion to their levels in the arterial blood (Figure 4). Whether the same occurs in diabetic ketoacidosis is still uncertain. Studies by Kety and his associates (Kety et al., 1948; Kety, 1957) revealed no significant cerebral arteriovenous difference for total ketones in diabetic acidosis or coma, but more recent studies by Gottstein et al. (in press) provide evidence of some cerebral uptake of ketone bodies in diabetic acidosis. It is possible that the hyperglycemia and reduced cerebral metabolic rate present in diabetic acidosis complicate the unequivocable demonstration of cerebral ketone body utilization.

RELATIONSHIP OF CEREBRAL KETONE UTILIZATION TO DEPENDENCE ON GLUCOSE The finding that the brain can and does utilize ketone bodies under certain circumstances is not necessarily in conflict with earlier observations that neither D-β-hydroxybutyrate nor acetoacetate can restore normal cerebral function and metabolism in hypoglycemia (Kety, 1957; Sokoloff, 1972). In all the studies demonstrating cerebral ketone utilization, glucose consumption may have been reduced but was still present to an appreciable degree. There is no evidence that ketone bodies can completely replace glucose. Indeed, there is evidence to the contrary; in the perfused rat brain complete replacement of glucose with D-β-hydroxybutyrate results in just as rapid deterioration of cerebral functional and metabolic activities as observed with complete removal of all substrate (Sloviter, personal communication). A possible explanation for the inability of ketone bodies to substitute for glucose completely may be in the pathway of their metabolism. As can be seen in Figure 2, D-β-hydroxybutyrate must first be converted to acetoacetate, and acetoacetate is further metabolized by displacing the succinyl moiety of succinyl CoA to form acetoacetyl CoA. In its usual pathway of metabolism succinyl CoA hydrolysis is normally coupled to GTP synthesis, and GTP has important functions in tissue metabolism, including protein synthesis and gluconeogenesis. Recent findings also suggest that cyclic GMP, which is formed from GTP, may play a role in mediating cholinergic synaptic transmission (Ferrendelli et al., 1970). There must also be sufficient succinyl CoA to sustain continued acetoacetate utilization. Indeed, Itoh and Quastel (1970) have found that the utilization of acetoacetate by brain slices is accelerated by the inclusion of glucose in the incubation medium, probably as a result of increased succinyl CoA levels. It is possible, therefore, that exclusive dependence on the utilization of ketones depletes the succinyl CoA and also the GTP levels in brain and that some glucose utilization is required to maintain them at adequate levels.

Enzymes of ketone utilization in the brain

ENZYMATIC STEPS IN PATHWAY OF KETONE UTILIZATION The pathways and enzymes of ketone utilization are illustrated in Figure 2. Two enzymes, 3-ketoacid CoA-transferase and acetoacetyl CoA thiolase, are required to metabolize acetoacetate to acetyl CoA, the first intermediate in common with the pathway of glucose metabolism and the one which enters the tricarboxylic acid cycle for ultimate oxidation to CO_2 and water. The utilization of the other ketone body, D-β-hydroxybutyrate (3-hydroxybutyrate) requires one additional enzyme, D-β-hydroxybutyrate dehydrogenase, to oxidize it to acetoacetate which is then metabolized as above. All three reactions are freely reversible.

The three enzymes are widely distributed in mammalian tissues (Lehninger et al., 1960; Krebs et al., 1971; Dierks-Ventling, 1971; Page et al., 1971; Tildon and Sevdalian, 1972) although the D-β-hydroxybutyrate dehydrogenase, which is present in highest amounts in the liver of the rat (Lehninger et al., 1960), is reported to be absent in the liver of ruminants (Nielsen and Fleischer, 1969). Also, the mammalian liver generally lacks the transferase (Mahler, 1953) and is, therefore, entirely incapable of metabolizing ketone bodies. It can, however, produce acetoacetate from acetoacetyl CoA and acetyl CoA that are formed in the course of fatty acid oxidation. Since it can produce them and not utilize them, the liver is the primary source of the ketone bodies in the blood, and its rate of production is enhanced with increasing fatty acid utilization. The D-β-hydroxybutyrate dehydrogenase in liver functions mainly in the reverse direction and converts the acetoacetate produced in the liver to D-β-hydroxybutyrate. Since the redox potential in the liver during fatty acid oxidation and the equilibrium constant at physiological pH probably favor this reverse direction, D-β-hydroxybutyrate is found in blood in severalfold higher concentrations than that of acetoacetate during naturally occurring ketosis (Owen et al., 1967; Krebs, 1971). It is, therefore, D-β-hydroxybutyrate that is predominantly utilized by the brain in ketotic states (Owen et al., 1967; Krebs et al., 1971).

DEVELOPMENTAL CHANGES IN ENZYME LEVELS The rise in cerebral oxygen consumption during postnatal development of the brain (Figure 1) reflects not only increased energy demand associated with the development of cerebral functional activity but also a concomitant rise in the levels of mitochondrial enzymes of oxidative metabolism. Most of these enzymes begin to rise shortly after birth, continue to rise throughout the period of brain maturation, and eventually level off at the normal adult level when the brain is mature. Some of these enzymes are included in the list in Table I. During the early rising phase the various mitochondrial enzymes increase more or less in proportion to one another, suggesting an increasing content of mitochondria in the developing brain. The proportions are not, however, maintained indefinitely. There are individual differences in the patterns of enzyme development, indicating that the regulation is not merely of the content of mitochondria but is also at the level of the individual enzymes. The enzymes specific to the pathway of ketone body utilization are among those that exhibit unique developmental patterns in brain. Figure 5 compares the postnatal developmental patterns of rat brain cytochrome oxidase, an enzyme of the electron transport chain, and D-β-hydroxybutyrate dehydrogenase, which is associated with the inner mitochondrial membrane and catalyzes the first step in the utilization of ketone bodies. The cytochrome oxidase exhibits the pattern typical of most mitochondrial oxidative enzymes. The D-β-hydroxybutyrate dehydrogenase rises at first proportionately with the cytochrome oxidase, but at 20 to 25 days of age, when the cytochrome oxidase level stabilizes and becomes constant, the dehydrogenase declines again and gradually reverts in adulthood almost to the low levels present at birth (Klee and Sokoloff, 1967; Pull and McIlwain, 1971; Krebs et al., 1971; Dahlquist et al., 1972). The second enzyme of the pathway of ketone body utilization, 3-ketoacid transferase, shows an almost identical pattern of development (Figure 3) (Krebs et al., 1971; Tildon et al., 1971). The third enzyme of the pathway, acetoacetyl CoA thiolase, follows an entirely different pattern; it is already maximal at birth, remains constant during the first 30 days of life, and then gradually declines to a level in adulthood about two-thirds that of infancy (Krebs et al., 1971; Dierks-Ventling and Cone, 1971a). It must be noted, however, that in contrast to the dehydrogenase and transferase, which serve only the pathways of ketone body metabolism, the thiolase functions in other metabolic processes as well, e.g. fatty acid oxidation, cholesterol biosynthesis, etc. It is clear that the enzymes, which are unique to the metabolism of ketone bodies, are also uniquely regulated during the postnatal maturation of the brain.

REGULATION OF ENZYMES OF KETONE UTILIZATION IN BRAIN   Throughout the life-span, whenever the ketone body concentrations rise in the blood, regardless of cause, the brain switches, at least in part, from almost complete dependence on glucose to the utilization of the ketone bodies in more or less proportion to their levels in the arterial blood (Krebs et al., 1971). In the adult this switch is accomplished without any change in the amounts of the enzymes of ketone utilization in the brain (Krebs, 1971), nor is any required. In the adult rat brain the maximum velocities of all three enzymes are comparable; the thiolase is present in slight excess, and the transferase appears to be slightly rate limiting (Figure 3) (Krebs, 1971). The maximum possible rate of acetyl CoA formation from either D-β-hydroxybutyrate or acetoacetate can be estimated to be about 80 μmole per 100 g of tissue per minute. Since normal cerebral glucose consumption generates approximately 60 μmole of acetyl CoA per 100 g per minute, the enzymes of ketone utilization are present in sufficient amounts in adult brain to satisfy its energy needs from ketone bodies. Maximal rates are rarely if ever achieved, however, because the concentrations of ketone bodies probably never rise high enough to saturate the enzymes. Control of ketone utilization in adult brain is achieved, therefore, merely by the simplest regulatory mechanism of all: substrate concentration and degree of saturation of the enzymes of ketone utilization.

Regulation of cerebral ketone utilization is, however, considerably more complex during postnatal maturation of the brain. Regulation by substrate concentration occurs (Figure 4), but, in addition, there are profound changes in the levels of the D-β-hydroxybutyrate dehydrogenase and the 3-ketoacid transferase (Figure 3) (Klee and Sokoloff, 1967; Krebs et al., 1971). Hormonal influences undoubtedly play a part. Thyroxine, for example, which accelerates the postnatal development of cerebral oxidative metabolism (Figure 1) also advances the developmental pattern of D-β-hydroxybutyrate dehydrogenase (Figure 6) (Grave et al., 1973). This effect of

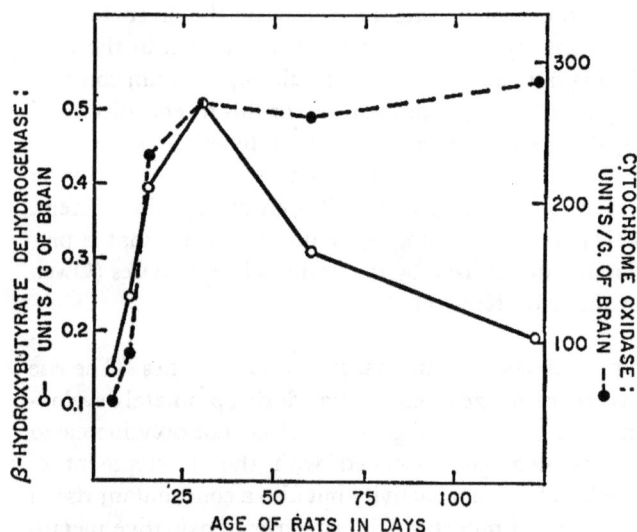

FIGURE 5   Changes in activities of the mitochondrial enzymes, cytochrome oxidase and D-β-hydroxybutyrate dehydrogenase, in rat brain during postnatal maturation. From Klee and Sokoloff (1967).

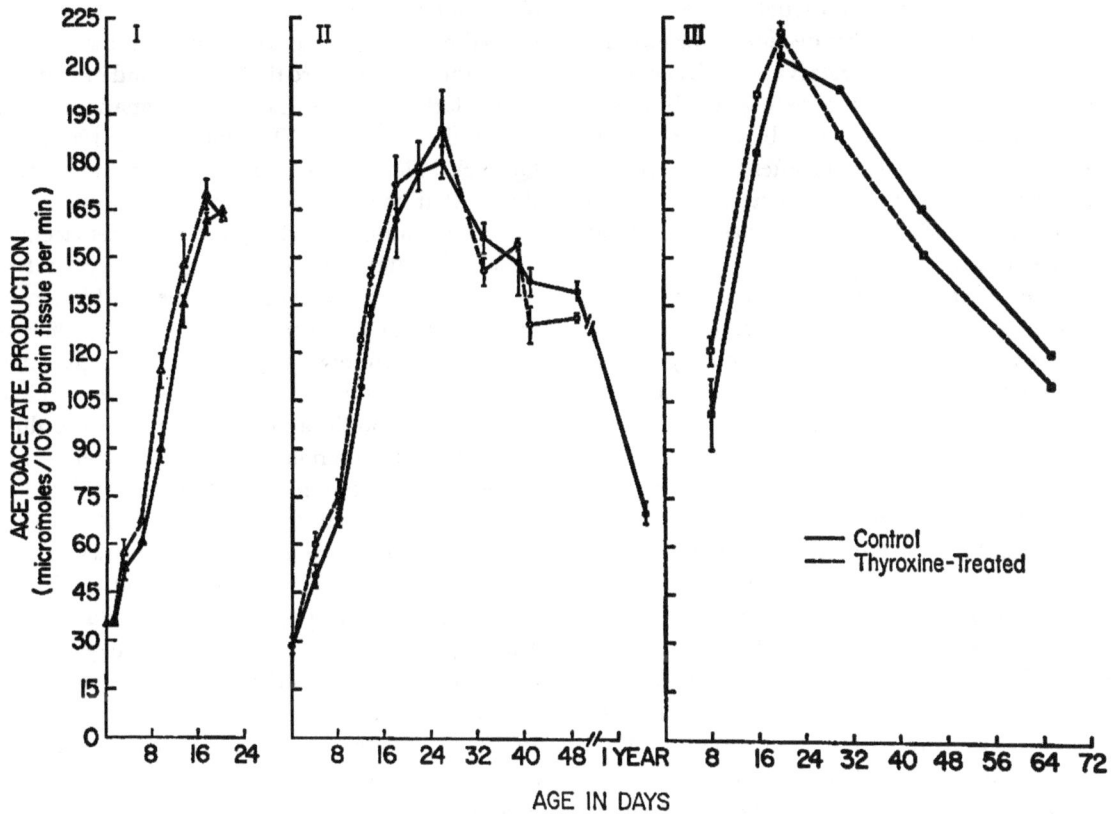

FIGURE 6 Effects of the administration of L-thyroxine from birth on the postnatal development of D-β-hydroxybutyrate dehydrogenase activity in rat brain. Series I, II, and II refer to 3 different series of experiments with different schedules of thyroxine administration. In Series I the experimental animals received 10 μg of sodium L-throxine intraperitoneally on the first day of age and every 48 hr thereafter; control littermates received only the solvent that consisted of 0.1 ml of 0.005 N NaOH–0.45% (w/v) NaCl. At this dosage there was significant impairment of brain and total body growth. In Series II, the same dosage was given but at 72 hr intervals, and no effects on brain and body growth were observed. In Series III, the dosage schedule used in Series I was followed for the first 4 doses and then switched to the dosage schedule of Series II. In all three series, the acceleration of the changes in the enzyme activity caused by thyroxine was statistically significant ($P < 0.05$) on the basis of multivariate profile analysis. From Grave et al. (1973).

thyroid hormones is not specific for the enzymes of ketone utilization; they have similar effects on other oxidative enzymes (Sokoloff, 1971). Of particular interest is the temporal relationship between the blood ketone levels and the enzyme activities in brain. The developmental patterns of the dehydrogenase and transferase in brain closely follow the changes in the concentrations of their substrates, D-β-hydroxybutyrate and acetoacetate, respectively, in blood. With the onset of suckling, for example, the newborn rat develops a marked ketosis as a result of the ketogenic nature of the maternal milk diet (Figure 3). This is followed by a rise in the dehydrogenase and the transferase levels in brain (Figure 3). When in the normal course of events the animals are weaned onto a standard diet at 20 to 25 days of age, the ketosis dissipates, and this is then followed by a decline in the levels of the enzymes in the brain. The enzymes of ketone body utilization in the developing brain appear, therefore, to be closely adjusted to the levels of available substrate. The mechanism of this adjustment is unknown. Whether it reflects induction of enzyme synthesis by the ketosis, protection of the enzymes from degradation by saturation with their substrates (Schimke, 1969), or merely a fortuitous correlation remains to be determined. There is controversial evidence to suggest that ketosis may play a direct role in the mechanism of the enzyme changes in the brain. In one study, maternal starvation and fasting at birth, which cause premature ketosis in the fetus and newborn animal, were found to accelerate the rise of 3-hydroxybutyrate dehydrogenase activity in the brains of fetal and neonatal rats (Thaler, 1972), but in another study no such effects were observed (Dahlquist et al., 1972). Prolongation of ketosis, following weaning by starvation or fat feeding, delays the decline in brain dehydrogenase activity that normally occurs at this time of life (Smith et al., 1969; Pull and McIlwain, 1971), and premature weaning onto a high-carbohydrate diet has been reported to initiate an earlier decline in the enzyme level (Smith et al., 1969). Neither starvation (Krebs et al., 1971; Tildon et al., 1971) nor fat feeding (Krebs et al., 1971; Dierks-Ventling and Cone, 1971b) appear to alter brain transferase activity at any age after birth although a maternal high-fat diet has been reported to increase both the transferase and thiolase activities of fetal rat brain (Dierks-Ventling, 1971).

Recent studies of the properties of the D-β-hydroxybutyrate dehydrogenase suggest an additional factor that may play a role in the changes in the activity of this enzyme during postnatal development of the brain. This enzyme exists in situ firmly bound to the inner mitochondrial membrane. It has recently been solubilized by cholate treatment of mitochondria isolated from weanling rat brain and partially purified by salt fractionation (Fitzgerald et al., 1973). The activity of the partially purified enzyme exhibits an absolute dependence on the presence of phospholipid extracted from the mitochondria. The active phospholipid has been tentatively identified as a lecithin, and some other phospholipids, such as lysolecithin, phosphatidylinositol and cardiolipin, are inhibitory. Egg lecithin and beef heart lecithin can substitute for the endogenous phospholipid; but far greater concentrations on the basis of phosphate content are required to achieve activities equivalent to those observed with the endogenous phospholipid. Heart (Fleischer et al., 1966) and liver (Gotterer, 1967) D-β-hydroxybutyrate dehydrogenase have been found to have similar properties. The exact identity of the lecithin and its mechanism of activation of the enzyme are unknown, but it cannot be neglected as a possible factor in the regulation of the enzyme's activity. Indeed, we can conceive of the possibility that the changes in D-β-hydroxybutyrate dehydrogenase activity in the brain during postnatal development and their relationship to suckling and weaning may reflect not so much regulation of the amount of enzyme as the influence of changes in the levels of the active phospholipid.

Summary

The mammalian brain undergoes a major portion of its maturation in early postnatal life. During this period there are marked changes in a number of enzyme activities, including those involved in cerebral energy metabolism. Indeed, it has now become clear that the regulation of cerebral energy metabolism occurs all through life and confers hitherto unrecognized flexibility to the brain in its choice of substrates for oxidative metabolism. The normal adult brain utilizes glucose almost exclusively as the substrate for its energy metabolism, but, contrary to previous beliefs, it is not obligatorily limited only to glucose. It has been known from studies with brain slices in vitro that mature and immature brain, particularly the latter, have the enzymatic machinery to oxidize ketone bodies (Drahota et al., 1965; Itoh and Quastel, 1970). Recent studies in man and animals have shown that the brain in vivo turns in special circumstances to D-β-hydroxybutyrate and acetoacetate as its main substrates. The ketone bodies serve not only as sources of energy derived from their oxidation to CO_2 and water but also contribute carbon residues to constituents of brain normally dependent on glucose metabolism, e.g. phospholipids and cholesterol (Spitzer and Weng, 1972) and the amino acids, glutamate, glutamine, aspartate and γ-aminobutyric acid (Cremer, 1971).

Ketone utilization in adult brain is regulated entirely by the supply of substrate brought to it in the arterial blood. The concentration of ketone bodies in the blood is normally very low in the adult, and cerebral ketone utilization is then negligible. In ketotic states caused, for example, by starvation or high-fat ketogenic diets, the brain utilizes ketone bodies in almost direct proportion to their concentrations in the arterial blood (Krebs, 1971). Their rate of utilization may then exceed that of glucose, although there is reason to doubt that they can replace glucose completely.

Significant rates of cerebral ketone utilization are normal in early postnatal life, and, contrary to the situation in adult life, regulation is achieved not only by substrate supply but also by modification of the levels of enzyme activity. The newborn is slightly hypoglycemic and becomes ketotic as a result of the high-fat content of maternal milk. The activities of two key enzymes of ketone utilization progressively increase in the brain throughout the suckling period and then decline again following weaning and the disappearance of the diet-induced ketosis. Whether or not the enzymes can be artificially induced by ketosis is still uncertain as regards early life, but clearly it does not occur in adult life. Whether the regulation of the activities of the enzymes in early life is achieved by changes in enzyme synthesis, enzyme degradation, or modification of catalytic activity of a constant level of enzyme molecules remains to be determined.

The brain is, therefore, not the inflexible, selective organ it was once thought to be but shares with many other organs the capacity to adapt to changes in its nutrient supply. Glucose still appears to be its substrate of choice and may even be essential to some degree, but when the brain's glucose supply becomes endangered and/or ketone bodies become more available, it can turn to ketone bodies for a significant fraction of its energy supply.

REFERENCES

BALÁZS, R., S. KOVACS, P. TEICHGRÄBER, W. A. COCKS, and J. T. EAYRS, 1968. Biochemical effects of thyroid deficiency on the developing brain. *J. Neurochem.* 15:1335–1349.

CREMER, J., 1971. Incorporation of label from D-β-hydroxy-[^{14}C]butyrate and [3-^{14}C]acetoacetate into amino acids in rat brain in vivo. *Biochem. J.* 122:135–138.

DAHLQUIST, G., U. PERSSON, and B. PERSSON, 1972. The activity of D-β-hydroxybutyrate dehydrogenase in fetal, infant, and adult rat brain and the influence of starvation. *Biol. Neonate* 20:40–52.

DIERKS-VENTLING, C., 1971. Prenatal induction of ketone-body enzymes in the rat. *Biol. Neonate* 19:423–433.

DIERKS-VENTLING, C., and A. L. CONE, 1971a. Acetoacetyl-coenzyme A thiolase in brain, liver, and kidney during maturation of the rat. *Science* 172:380–382.

DIERKS-VENTLING, C., and A. L. CONE, 1971b. Ketone body enzymes in mammalian tissues. *J. Biol. Chem.* 246:5533–5534.

DRAHOTA, Z., P. HAHN, J. MOUREK, and M. TROJANOVA, 1965. The effect of acetoacetate on oxygen consumption of brain slices from infant and adult rats. *Physiol. Bohemoslav.* 14:134–136.

DYMSZA, H. A., D. M. CZAJKA, and S. A. MILLER, 1964. Influence of artificial diet on weight gain and body composition of the neonatal rat. *J. Nutr.* 84:100–106.

EAYRS, J. T., 1964. Endocrine influence on cerebral development. *Arch. Biol. (Liege)* 75:529–565.

FAZEKAS, J. F., F. B. GRAVES, and R. W. ALMAN, 1951. The influence of the thyroid on cerebral metabolism. *Endocrinology* 48:169–174.

FERRENDELLI, J. A., A. L. STEINER, D. B. McDOUGAL, JR., and D. M. KIPNIS, 1970. The effect of oxotremorine and atropine on cGMP and cAMP levels in mouse cerebral cortex and cerebellum. *Biochem. Biophys. Res. Commun.* 41:1061–1067.

FITZGERALD, G. G., E. E. KAUFMAN, and L. SOKOLOFF, 1973. Partial purification and properties of rat brain D-β-hydroxybutyrate dehydrogenase, *Fed. Proc.* 32:563 (abs).

FLEISCHER, B., A. CASU, and S. FLEISCHER, 1966. Release of β-hydroxybutyric apodehydrogenase from beef heart mitochondria by the action of phospholipase A. *Biochem. Biophys. Res. Commun.* 24:189–194.

GARCIA ARGIZ, C. A., J. M. PASQUINI, B. KAPLUN, and C. J. GOMEZ, 1967. Hormonal regulation of brain development. II. Effect of neonatal thyroidectomy on succinate dehydrogenase and other enzymes in developing cerebral cortex and cerebellum of the rat. *Brain Res.* 6:635–646.

GOTTERER, G. S., 1967. Rat liver D-β-hydroxybutyrate dehydrogenase. II. Lipid requirement. *Biochemistry* 6:2147–2152.

GOTTSTEIN, U., K. HELD, W. MÜLLER, and W. BERGHOFF, 1972. *Research on the Cerebral Circulation. Fifth International Salzburg Conference, 1970,* J. S. Meyer, M. Reivich, and H. Lechner, eds. Springfield, Ill.: Charles C. Thomas, (in press).

GRAVE, G. D., S. SATTERTHWAITE, C. KENNEDY, and L. SOKOLOFF, 1973. Accelerated postnatal development of D(-)-β-hydroxybutyrate dehydrogenase (EC 1.1.1.30) activity in the brain in hyperthyroidism. *J. Neurochem.* 20:495–502.

HAMBURGH, M., and L. B. FLEXNER, 1957. Physiological differentiation during morphogenesis. XXI. Effect of hypothyroidism and hormone therapy on enzyme activities of the developing cerebral cortex of the rat. *J. Neurochem.* 1:279–288.

HAWKINS, R. A., D. H. WILLIAMSON, and H. A. KREBS, 1971.

Ketone-body utilization by adult and suckling rat brain in vivo. *Biochem. J.* 122:13–18.

ITOH, T., and J. H. QUASTEL, 1970. Acetoacetate metabolism in infant and adult rat brain in vitro. *Biochem. J.* 116:641–655.

KETY, S. S., 1957. The general metabolism of the brain in vivo. In *Metabolism of the Nervous System,* D. Richter, ed. London: Pergamon Press, pp. 221–237.

KETY, S. S., B. D. POLIS, C. S. NADLER, and C. F. SCHMIDT, 1948. The blood flow and oxygen consumption of the human brain in diabetic acidosis and coma. *J. Clin. Invest.* 27:500–510.

KIZER, D. E., and T. A. McCOY, 1960. Phosphomannose isomerase activity in a spectrum of normal and malignant rat tissues. *Proc. Soc. Exp. Biol. Med.* 103:772–774.

KLEE, C. B., and L. SOKOLOFF, 1964. Mitochondrial differences in mature and immature brain. Influence on rate of amino acid incorporation into protein and responses to thyroxine. *J. Neurochem.* 11:709–716.

KLEE, C. B., and L. SOKOLOFF, 1967. Changes in D(-)-β-hydroxybutyric dehydrogenase activity during brain maturation in the rat. *J. Biol. Chem.* 242:3880–3883.

KOSHLAND, JR., D. E., 1970. The molecular basis for enzyme regulation. In *The Enzymes,* Vol. I, 3rd Ed., P. D. Boyer, ed. New York: Academic Press, pp. 341–396.

KREBS, H. A., D. H. WILLIAMSON, M. W. BATES, M. A. PAGE, and R. A. HAWKINS, 1971. The role of ketone bodies in caloric homeostasis. *Adv. Enzyme Regul.* 9:387–409.

LEHNINGER, A. L., H. C. SUDDUTH, and J. B. WISE, 1960. D-β-hydroxybutyric dehydrogenase of mitochondria. *J. Biol. Chem.* 235:2450–2455.

MAHLER, H. R., 1953. Role of coenzyme A in fatty acid metabolism. *Fed. Proc.* 12:694–702.

McILWAIN, H., 1971. Types of metabolic adaptation in the brain. *Essays in Biochemistry* 7:127–158.

MICHELS, R., J. CASON, and L. SOKOLOFF, 1963. Thyroxine: Effects on amino acid incorporation into protein in vivo. *Science* 140:1417–1418.

MURTHY, M. R. V., and D. A. RAPPOPORT, 1963. Biochemistry of the developing rat brain. III. Mitochondrial oxidation of citrate and isocitrate and associated phosphorylation. *Biochim. Biophys. Acta* 74:328–339.

NIELSEN, N. C., and S. FLEISCHER, 1969. β-Hydroxybutyrate dehydrogenase: Lack in ruminant liver mitochondria. *Science* 166:1017–1019.

OWEN, O. E., A. P. MORGAN, H. G. KEMP, J. M. SULLIVAN, M. G. HERRERA, and G. F. CAHILL, 1967. Brain metabolism during fasting. *J. Clin. Invest.* 46:1589–1595.

PAGE, M. A., H. A. KREBS, and D. H. WILLIAMSON, 1971. Activities of enzymes of ketone-body utilization in brain and other tissues of suckling rats. *Biochem. J.* 121:49–53.

PASQUINI, J. M., B. KAPLUN, C. A. GARCIA ARGIZ, and C. J. GOMEZ, 1967. Hormonal regulation of brain development. I. The effect of neonatal thyroidectomy upon nucleic acids, protein, and two enzymes in developing cerebral cortex and cerebellum of the rat. *Brain Res.* 6:621–634.

PERSSON, B., G. SETTERGREN, and G. DAHLQUIST, 1972. Cerebral arteriovenous difference of acetoacetate and D-β-hydroxybutyrate in children. *Acta Paediatr. Scand.* 61:273–278.

PULL, I., and H. McILWAIN, 1971. 3-hydroxybutyrate dehydrogenase of rat brain on dietary change and during maturation. *J. Neurochem.* 18:1163–1165.

RASKIN, N. H., and L. SOKOLOFF, 1970. Alcohol dehydrogenase activity in rat brain and liver. *J. Neurochem.* 17:1677–1687.

SCHIMKE, R. T., 1969. On the roles of synthesis and degradation in regulation of enzyme levels in mammalian tissues. In *Current Topics in Cellular Regulation*, B. Horecker and E. R. Stadtman, eds. New York: Academic Press, pp. 77–124.

SCHMIDT, M. J., and G. A. ROBISON, 1972. The effect of neonatal thyroidectomy on the development of the adenosine 3′,5′-monophosphate system in the rat brain. *J. Neurochem.* 19:937–947.

SCHWARK, W. S., R. L. SINGHAL, and G. M. LING, 1972. Metabolic control mechanisms in mammalian systems. Regulation of key glycolytic enzymes in developing brain during experimental cretinism. *J. Neurochem.* 19:1171–1182.

SLOVITER, H. A., and T. KAMIMOTO, 1970. The isolated, perfused brain preparation metabolizes mannose but not maltase. *J. Neurochem.* 17:1109–1111.

SLOVITER, H. A., P. SHIMKIN, and K. SUHARA, 1966. Glycerol as substrate for brain metabolism. *Nature (Lond.)* 210:1334–1336.

SLOVITER, H. A., and K. SUHARA, 1967. A brain-infusion method for demonstrating utilization of glycerol by rabbit brain in vivo. *J. Appl. Physiol.* 23:792–797.

SMITH, A. L., H. S. SATTERTHWAITE, and L. SOKOLOFF, 1969. Changes in brain D(-)-β-hydroxybutyrate dehydrogenase activity with development and during adaptation to altered substrate supply. *Proc. Second Int. Meeting Int. Soc. Neurochem. Abstr.*, R. Paoletti, R. Fumagalli, and C. Galli, eds. Milan, Italy: Tamburini Editore, p. 371.

SOKOLOFF, L., 1968. Role of mitochondria in the stimulation of protein synthesis by thyroid hormones. In *Some Regulatory Mechanisms for Protein Synthesis in Mammalian Cells*, Proc. of Third Kettering Symposium, 1968, A. Pietro, M. R. Lamborg, and F. T. Kenney, eds. New York: Academic Press, pp. 345–367.

SOKOLOFF, L., 1970. The mechanism of action of thyroid hormones on protein synthesis and its relationship to the differences in sensitivities of mature and immature brain. In *Protein Metabolism of the Nervous System*, A. Lajtha, ed. New York: Plenum Press, pp. 367–382.

SOKOLOFF, L., 1971. Action of thyroid hormones. In *Handbook of Neurochemistry*, Vol. 7, Part B, A. Lajtha, ed. New York: Plenum Press, pp. 525–549.

SOKOLOFF, L., 1972. Circulation and energy metabolism of the brain. In *Basic Neurochemistry*, R. W. Albers, B. Agranoff, R. Katzman, and G. J. Siegel, eds. Boston: Little, Brown, pp. 299–325.

SOKOLOFF, L., and S. KAUFMAN, 1961. Thyroxine stimulation of amino acid incorporation into protein. *J. Biol. Chem.* 236:795–803.

SOKOLOFF, L., P. A. ROBERTS, M. M. JANUSKA, and J. E. KLINE, 1968. Mechanisms of stimulation of protein synthesis by thyroid hormones in vivo. *Proc. Nat. Acad. Sci. USA* 60:652–659.

SPITZER, J. J., and J. J. WENG, 1972. Removal and utilization of ketone bodies by the brain of newborn puppies. *J. Neurochem.* 19:2169–2173.

SWAIMAN, K. F., J. M. DALEIDEN, and R. N. WOLFE, 1970. The effect of food deprivation on enzyme activity in developing brain. *J. Neurochem.* 17:1387–1391.

TATA, J. R., and C. C. WIDNELL, 1966. Ribonucleic acid synthesis during the early action of thyroid hormones. *Biochem. J.* 98:604–620.

THALER, M. M., 1972. Effects of starvation on normal development of β-hydroxybutyrate dehydrogenase activity in fetal and newborn rat brain. *Nature New Biol.* 236:140–141.

TILDON, J. T., A. L. CONE, and M. CORNBLATH, 1971. Coenzyme A transferase activity in rat brain. *Biochem. Biophys. Res. Commun.* 43:225–231.

TILDON, J. T., and D. A. SEVDALIAN, 1972. CoA transferase in the brain and other mammalian tissues. *Arch. Biochem. Biophys.* 148:382–390.

VALCANA, T., and P. S. TIMIRAS, 1969. Effect of hypothyroidism on ionic metabolism and Na-K activated ATP phosphohydrolase activity in the developing rat brain. *J. Neurochem.* 16:935–943.

VOLPE, J. J., and Y. KISHIMOTO, 1972. Fatty acid synthetase of brain: Development, influence of nutritional and hormonal factors and comparison with liver enzyme. *J. Neurochem.* 19:737–753.

www.ingramcontent.com/pod-product-compliance
Lightning Source LLC
Chambersburg PA
CBHW061754210326
41518CB00036B/2450